'*Mindful Little Yogis* is an excellent, user-friendly book full of fun, practical ideas for children and young adults with special needs. As a movement therapist I particularly enjoyed the yoga postures and the Lazy Eight Breathing technique. The STAR model that divides each chapter is a very clever idea, reminding readers to be mindful throughout. A must-have book for anyone supporting individuals or groups.'

– Cathy Underwood, Yoga and Inclusive Movement
Therapist, SYT Yoga Alliance Professionals, UK

'*Mindful Little Yogis* is an essential guide to your daily practice, whether you are a parent, an educator, or carer in the field of special needs. It is written in a user-friendly way, with a clear understanding of what the students need. The techniques make you want to experiment with mindfulness and yoga right away.'

– Mikaela Shalders, Paediatric Occupational
Therapist and Sensory Integration Specialist

'An essential book to own if you would like to be guided through, step-by-step, some extremely practical and mindfully structured lessons on your well-being journey, in a holistic way. You can trust that this book is going to guide you through your journey and that you will be able to spread the power of shining from within.'

– Timea Viragh, SENCO Teacher and Yoga Teacher

of related interest

Asanas for Autism and Special Needs
Yoga to Help Children with their Emotions, Self-Regulation and Body Awareness
Shawnee Thornton Hardy
ISBN 978 1 84905 988 6
eISBN 978 1 78450 059 7

The Go Yogi! Card Set
50 Everyday Yoga Poses for Calm, Happy, Healthy Kids
Emma Hughes
Illustrated by John Smisson
ISBN 978 1 84819 370 3

Sitting on a Chicken
The Best (Ever) 52 Yoga Games to Teach in Schools
Michael Chissick
Illustrated by Sarah Peacock
ISBN 978 1 84819 325 3
eISBN 978 0 85701 280 7

Mindful Little Yogis

Self-Regulation Tools to Empower Kids with Special Needs to Breathe and Relax

NICOLA HARVEY

Illustrations by John Smisson

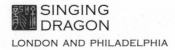

SINGING
DRAGON
LONDON AND PHILADELPHIA

First published in 2018
by Singing Dragon
an imprint of Jessica Kingsley Publishers
73 Collier Street
London N1 9BE, UK
and
400 Market Street, Suite 400
Philadelphia, PA 19106, USA

www.singingdragon.com

Library of Congress Cataloging in Publication Data
Names: Harvey, Nicola, author.
Title: Mindful little yogis : self-regulation tools to empower kids with
   special needs to breathe and relax / Nicola Harvey ; illustrations by John
   Smisson.
Description: London ; Philadelphia : Singing Dragon, [2018] | Includes
   bibliographical references and index.
Identifiers: LCCN 2018003163 | ISBN 9781848194045 (alk. paper)
Subjects: LCSH: Self-control in children. | Breathing exercises. | Hatha
   yoga. | Relaxation--Therapeutic use. | Behavior modification. |
   Mindfulness (Psychology) | Children with disabilities--Care.
Classification: LCC BF723.S25 H37 2018 | DDC 155--dc23 LC
record available at https://lccn.loc.gov/2018003163

British Library Cataloguing in Publication Data
A CIP catalogue record for this book is available from the British Library

ISBN 978 1 84819 404 5
eISBN 978 0 85701 360 6

Printed and bound in Great Britain

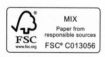

Contents

Part III: Relax

Part IV: Final Reflections

Part V: Resources

Acknowledgements

I am incredibly grateful and humbled to have been given the opportunity to create *Mindful Little Yogis*.

This book started as a simple idea from my blog to help children with special needs become the best versions of themselves. It has, however, taken on a life of its own, and writing this has carried me through a creative journey of hope, perseverance, joy and inspiration. I have many people to thank for making this possible.

I would like to thank the team at Singing Dragon Publishers and Jessica Kingsley, especially Sarah Hamlin, who saw the potential in the initial idea, and helped shape my vision into a reality. I am also thankful to John Smisson, Bonnie Craig, Victoria Peters and Rosamund Bird for their efforts and professionalism during the creation of *Mindful Little Yogis*.

Over the years I have been lucky enough to work with and learn from some amazing children, therapists, teachers, teaching assistants, mindfulness practitioners, parents, yogis and special needs professionals who have inspired me to write this book. Each of whom has shown that by adopting a flexible, resilient and empathetic attitude, every child can be helped and deserves a chance to shine.

For my close family's love and support over the years, I'd like to thank Joan, Basil, Andrea, Nathaniel, Tiana and Bailey. Without them, I would not be the person I am today. And thanks also to Julia, Elena, Juliet, Liz, Grace and Celia – friends who have become family.

Lastly, I would like to thank you for purchasing *Mindful Little Yogis* and for sharing my vision to nurture and empower children from all walks of life. I hope the self-regulation tools and mindfulness concepts in this book enable the children in your life to find a sense of inner peace. **Namaste** ♥

Disclaimer

The contents of *Mindful Little Yogis* including but not limited to the text, illustrations, diagrams, tables, resources and other material are for informational purposes only. The purpose of this book is to raise awareness of using mindfulness and self-regulation tools to support children from all walks of life and all abilities, particularly those with special needs.

It is always advisable to seek the advice of a qualified and experienced medical professional or therapist with any specific questions you may have regarding a medical condition, mental health issue or treatment plan. *Mindful Little Yogis* is not a substitute for professional medical advice, diagnosis or treatment. Whilst these breathing activities can be completed at any time and in any suitable space, children's specific needs, safety and emotional well-being are paramount so please be mindful and act responsibly at all times.

With all the activities contained within *Mindful Little Yogis*, please ensure you check the requirements, therapeutic benefits and developmental skills of each activity carefully to ensure children have the most appropriate tools and are as comfortable as possible. The Developmental Skills Glossary in Part V provides further clarification.

To reiterate, the activities contained within this book are for guidance purposes only and do not act as a replacement for medical treatment. Consult a medical professional for advice if children or adults experience health concerns, particularly of a respiratory or cardiovascular nature, or for clarification on the suitability of any breathing activities contained within this book.

Introduction

Mindful Little Yogis is an accessible tool for every parent, educator, therapist or individual with an interest in using mindfulness to nurture children's physical, mental and emotional well-being. This is a book to help the special kids in your life to find a sense of calm from within, a balanced outlook and a self-assured approach to experiencing life.

With the highs and lows of life's daily demands and pressures, getting through each day can be an incredibly overwhelming experience for children, especially for kids with special needs. A child with special needs views and experiences the world around them differently. To this end, it's our responsibility to teach kids mindfulness to help them calmly process experiences, recognise that it's okay to have feelings and celebrate their unique traits.

This is a book mindfully written by an experienced Special Needs Practitioner, who has worked with hundreds of children of all abilities in both mainstream and special needs settings and has seen first-hand how children requiring additional support find it difficult to fit in due to unrealistic expectations and innate misunderstandings of their unique personality traits. With an increase in the number of children experiencing mental health difficulties, there's been a distinctive rise in childhood anxiety, feelings of rejection, loneliness, depression and panic. To this end, many parents persevere and dig deep to ensure their child receives inclusive treatment, feels understood and is supported by professionals with their child's best interests at heart.

The activities in this book can be used to help kids in a variety of educational, therapeutic and casual settings. It's a practical book filled with simple breathing activities and handy self-regulation tools that can be slotted into mainstream or special needs classroom schedules as quick, mixed-ability, group sessions or 1:1 interventions to help settle heightened emotions. The resources marked with a ☯ are available to download and print for personal use from www.jkp.com/catalogue/book/97801848194045.

In the first chapter, readers are introduced to the world of special education needs (SEN) and how the ancient practice of yoga can teach 'special little yogis' to be in the present moment and learn how to process life's experiences. The second chapter takes a gradual approach to helping children breathe and shine from within using S.T.A.R. – Stop. Take a breath. And Relax. The third chapter shows readers an extensive range of yoga breathing (pranayama) activities to help children mindfully connect with their breath and gradually access a peaceful state of mind, emotional well-being and physiological awareness. The fourth chapter explores practical self-regulation tools to help children mindfully take ownership of their state and learn to 'go with the flow'. The fifth chapter shows us that textbook theory is very different to reality and provides positive strategies and ideas on how to help kids further if, when putting the activities into practice, things do not initially go to plan.

As you will see, *Mindful Little Yogis* has been written with the readers in mind: an essential text for anyone working or living with a child who needs support to feel grounded in the here and now. Although this book gives a range of useful tips and ideas, the book alone will not change your or children's well-being. This can only be done by putting the tools into practice yourself, and then modelling the activities to children, sharing these ideas with others and understanding the concept of mindfulness. By becoming a mindful yogi and experimenting with an open mind, readers are encouraged to explore the activities in this book, adapt if necessary and see what works best for the special little yogis in your life.

With continued practice and patience whilst using this book, readers will, over time, see a notable difference in children's emotional, mental and physical well-being, which can help them gradually grow into the best versions of themselves.

Chapter 1

Special Little Yogis

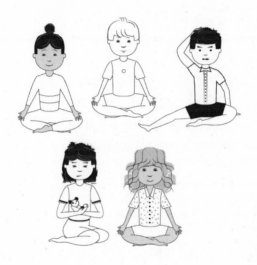

What is SEN?

Special educational needs (SEN) is a legal term used in the UK to describe a child or young person with a learning difficulty or disability who requires special provision to be made for him or her. Learning difficulties and disabilities can range from complex autism, dyslexia, dyscalculia, sensory processing disorder, cognitive development delay, Fragile X, attention deficit hyperactivity disorder (ADHD), profound and multiple learning disabilities (PMLD) and other neurological and development differences.

There are around one in five children with special needs in the UK (Ofsted, 2010), and many find it difficult to access age-related learning curriculums in educational facilities alongside their immediate peers.

A child with special needs may: find it hard to express him or herself or comprehend what someone else is saying; experience sensory or physical difficulties; need regular medical attention; or struggle with their behaviour, social interactions and emotions.

The *Special Educational Needs and Disability Code of Practice: 0 to 25 Years* (Department for Education, 2015) in England identifies four main areas where children with special needs may experience difficulty and with which they are required to receive adequate support.

- **Cognition and learning**: inclusive and differentiated support tailored towards children's ability to learn and process information, usually through individualised education plans detailing how children's additional learning needs can be accommodated in inclusive ways.

- **Social, emotional and mental health**: clear supportive structures, boundaries, calming strategies, empathy and safe spaces to feel a sense of belonging and appropriate channels to express themselves.

- **Communication and interaction**: differentiated communication, support with speech and language, particularly when providing visuals to help non-verbal children communicate and, depending on the children, ensuring low levels of sensory stimulus or distractions.

- **Sensory and/or physical needs**: accommodating children's specific sensory and physical needs may involve providing specialist therapy sessions and equipment, including walking frames, noise reduction headphones, sensory swings or fiddly toys.

It must be noted that every child is unique and has their own set of traits, behaviours and personal life experiences affecting how they view the world around them. Some children with special needs may require occasional assistance to access the curriculum and navigate their way through school routines, whereas others will need to be fully supported with specialist provision throughout their time in compulsory education and beyond. With this in mind, alongside the practical requirements of working or living with children with special needs, practitioners, guardians and carers need to exercise compassion, empathy and kindness, build trust and encourage children never to give up on themselves.

The Modern-Day Classroom

Year on year, an increasing number of children are identified with special needs, so the modern-day classroom is changing. In special schools and mainstream settings, educators are required to adopt a personalised approach towards teaching and learning, with inclusive practices, sensitivity towards students' differing needs, flexibility and patience.

Children can sense the way in which adults communicate with them and pick up on how they are treated by the adults in their lives. A passing comment from a teacher, friend or parent may seem harmless but could be perceived differently and potentially end up being detrimental for a child's mental and emotional well-being. Messages conveyed to children by adults create early belief systems that start to form their subconscious mind. This is their identity, their self-image and how they relate to their peers and connect with the world around them. Based on adult feedback, many children with special needs unknowingly compare themselves with more able peers and family members as they recognise subtle differences between their capabilities and their peers' and how people treat them. If this is not managed in a nurturing and inclusive manner by adults, it can result in feelings of rejection and loneliness, lack of self-esteem, confusion, anxiety or overwhelm. This is why it is imperative for all children to feel supported and treated with the kindness, integrity and sensitivity they deserve. Educators and therapists do this by: building rapport to develop a sense of trust; using tailored and multisensory methods to communicate; understanding children's specific traits, emotions and therapeutic needs; tapping into their learning styles; and introducing self-regulation to help them feel self-assured and empowered to take on each day. This is where mindfulness can help.

Mindful Yogis

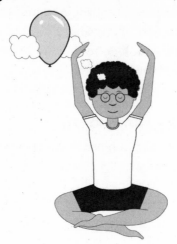

Mindfulness originates from Ancient Buddhism, Vedic traditions and other historic spiritual concepts. Jon Kabat-Zinn describes mindfulness as 'paying attention on purpose, without judgement, in the present moment' (2004: 4) whilst the *English Oxford Living Dictionaries* (Oxford University Press, 2015) defines mindfulness as a 'mental state achieved by focussing on one's awareness of the present moment, while calmly acknowledging and accepting one's feelings, thoughts and bodily sensations, used as a therapeutic technique'. More schools are bringing mindfulness into the modern-day classroom, and there are numerous benefits, particularly for children with special needs in busy educational settings. Mindfulness practice can help reduce anxiety, improve focus, increase cognitive flexibility, boost working memory, lower the recurrence of depression and enable better access to the curriculum (Sanger and Dorjee, 2015).

A yogi is a person who practices the principles of yoga. Yoga is a form of mindfulness and awareness of the whole body. Created over 5000 years ago by yogis seeking spiritual enlightenment, yoga consists of breathing (pranayama), physical poses (asana), meditation, relaxation and other activities to bring the mind, body and spirit into peaceful union. Traditional yogis see the practice of yoga as a way of embodying peace, kindness, unity and compassion into everything they do beyond the yoga mat. Yogis are encouraged to:

connect with themselves and others in a non-judgemental way; be still and present in each moment; and listen to their hearts and find their true paths in life.

Mindful yogis regularly focus on the breath, because everything starts with the breath. Every breath inhaled is a chance to allow life to flow through the body, let go of resistance and develop a sense of compassion. In the book, *Perfectly Imperfect*, Baron Baptiste suggests 'the breath is the key to unlocking your body's potential. Maintaining steady, rhythmic breathing is the single most important element of yoga practice' (2016: 35).

The next chapter profiles the S.T.A.R. model, which provides a framework in which children pause for a moment, connect to their breathing, gradually relax and find a sense of flow. This is followed by an extensive range of simple, mindful-breathing exercises to use with the S.T.A.R. model to empower little yogis to take control, calm their emotions and gain clarity of mind.

Chapter 2

Shine from Within

The S.T.A.R. model

The S.T.A.R. model consists of four stages: Stop. Take a breath. And. Relax. This is a step-by-step, visual mindfulness sequence that acts as a guide for children as they progress through the activities within this book. The diagram below provides key steps on how to communicate the use of self-regulation with children. Be sure to tailor the verbal input and language if required, and create visual picture cues to support children's understanding of S.T.A.R.

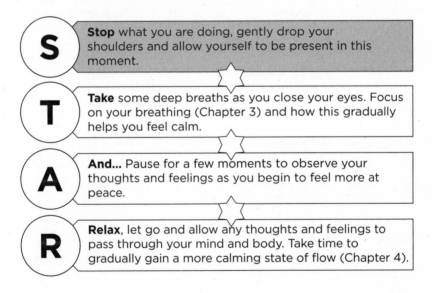

S — **Stop** what you are doing, gently drop your shoulders and allow yourself to be present in this moment.

T — **Take** some deep breaths as you close your eyes. Focus on your breathing (Chapter 3) and how this gradually helps you feel calm.

A — **And...** Pause for a few moments to observe your thoughts and feelings as you begin to feel more at peace.

R — **Relax**, let go and allow any thoughts and feelings to pass through your mind and body. Take time to gradually gain a more calming state of flow (Chapter 4).

S.T.A.R. is an essential development tool for children. Regular and diligent step-by-step practice of the activities contained within this book can create positive behavioural, mental, physical and emotional responses within children.

When a child frequently follows the S.T.A.R. model and participates in the mindfulness and self-regulation activities in this book, neuropathways are created in the brain. These neuropathways can gradually rewire the brain to create renewed ways of thinking, connecting to feelings and how the body physically reacts. This is neuroplasticity – the brain's ability to create new cells and adapt its formation based on the consistent habitual patterns, directed attention and regular stimuli it is exposed to. Although the responses generated will differ within the brain of a person with neurodevelopmental disabilities compared with a person with a neurotypical brain, with regular practice of the S.T.A.R. model (depending on children's specific needs, cognitive abilities and experience of self-regulation tools) neuroplasticity can instil positive and continual changes.

Stop

To initiate S.T.A.R. with children, calmly follow the guidance in part one (**stop**) of the diagram and ask children to gently drop the shoulders, pause to observe how they feel in their body and be present in the moment. This may take time, so adults need to hold the space with patience, calm and grounded reassurance before moving on to part two (**take a breath**). Whilst the S.T.A.R. is a simple and clear sequential process for children with special needs, in reality, if a child experiencing a meltdown is told to suddenly **stop** what they are doing (part one of S.T.A.R.), it may make things worse, as he or she could be consumed and caught up in that moment. If this is the case, give children time to move safely through their heightened emotions and then, when they appear settled, go straight to the practical mindful breathing exercises in Chapter 3.

Depending on the circumstances and the children in your life, things may change, so whilst using the S.T.A.R. model to incorporate mindfulness, be mindful of Master Yogi, Swami Sivananda's comments that it's acceptable for yogis to 'adapt, adjust and accommodate' where necessary. It's also important to have fun, so enjoy the process and be flexible to children's needs!

In the next chapter, we will explore the second part of the S.T.A.R. model by giving children the tools to calm the body and mind with a range of fun and simple mindful breathing activities.

Part I

Take a Breath

S	**Stop** what you are doing, gently drop your shoulders and allow yourself to be present in this moment.
T	**Take** some deep breaths as you close your eyes. Focus on your breathing (Chapter 3) and how this gradually helps you feel calm.
A	**And...** Pause for a few moments to observe your thoughts and feelings as you begin to feel more at peace.
R	**Relax**, let go and allow any thoughts and feelings to pass through your mind and body. Take time to gradually gain a more calming state of flow (Chapter 4).

Mindful Breathing

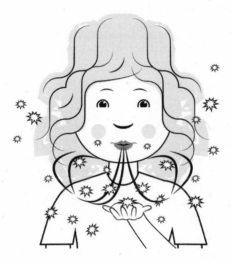

Be Conscious of the Breath

When children feel stressed, overwhelmed or anxious, the last thing on their mind is to consciously breathe. The breathing rhythm may therefore be at a shallow and faster pace, which can trigger or heighten panicked states, increase the heart rate, raise the blood pressure and reinforce disharmonious thoughts, feelings and behaviours.

When adults encourage children to consciously breathe and connect to the breath, it can make a huge difference. Breathing deeply and mindfully sends subtle messages between the brain and the parasympathetic nervous system to calm down, relax the bodily sensations and purify any busy thoughts.

Breathing is the core of mindfulness. Breathing takes place in the present moment. Continued focus on the breath can move us away from mind chatter and emotional upheaval, bringing us into a state of calm. Consciously breathing oxygen into the lungs means that cleansing energy is inhaled and circulated into the bloodstream. Exhaling carbon dioxide means that negative emotions and tension can be released into the air. Conscious breathing with a steady and continued inhale and exhale rhythm can bring a sense of flow into the body and mind and then balance emotions. When children learn how to connect and breathe mindfully, they become more present, grounded and self-assured.

The majority of the breathing activities contained in this chapter involve diaphragmatic or belly breathing. During diaphragmatic breathing, the abdomen expands when oxygen is deeply inhaled into the lungs, whilst the chest moves only slightly. This creates a more fulfilling and healthier process of self-regulating the mind and body from within.

The therapeutic benefits of diaphragmatic breathing are immense; it:

- balances, calms and connects the mind and body

- relieves stress, reduces anxiety and other mental/emotional conditions

- lowers the heart rate and blood pressure and improves blood circulation

- improves the cardiovascular system and reduces tension

- helps strengthen mental abilities, particularly abstract thoughts, working memory and introspection.

The mindful breathing activities in this chapter are categorised in the following sections:

- Breathe

- Sensory

- Animal breathing

- Shape breathing

- Sound

- Visualisation

- Body flow.

These activities are fun, simple and creative calming strategies to empower children to self-regulate and follow part two of the S.T.A.R. model from Chapter 2. Devised for children with special needs (although these activities benefit all children), each breathing tool lists:

- **therapeutic benefits,** in case adults would like children to achieve a particular state e.g. 'alert', 'mental clarity' or 'calm'

- **developmental skills,** with which children with special needs often need more guidance (see the Developmental Skills Glossary in Part V)

- **be mindful** notes for each breathing activity.

How to Initiate the Practice

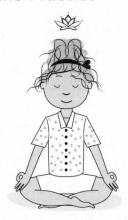

Find a comfortable space and inform the children that you will be introducing a deep-breathing activity to help them feel calm. With older children, depending on their level of understanding, inform them in more detail of the healing benefits of deep breathing on the mind and whole body, particularly in terms of focus and letting go of stress.

Choose one or two techniques from Section 1: Breathe for the children to do every day for a week, as the techniques in this section simply focus on the breath. With all the breathing exercises, initiate each activity by 'scaffolding': the adults should model or show each activity and then the children join in and copy the actions and instructions from the adults, eventually performing the breathing activities independently.

Once the children become familiar with the initial activities in Section 1: Breathe, show them how powerful and versatile their breath can be by using additional breathing exercises from this section. Then, when children are ready, progress through or dip into the other breathing sections in the rest of this chapter. Calming strategies are more effective when children tap into and explore their own interests, so feel free to adapt the exercises for children's preferences and any specific needs.

Please ensure children *do not lock and hold the breath* at any time, as this can ignite tension in the body and mind. Encourage a natural flow of the breath and simply pause to notice the sensation when this is required in any of the activities.

Carefully check the requirements, therapeutic benefits and developmental skills of each activity to ensure children have the most appropriate tools and are as comfortable as possible. Please note that these breathing activities can be completed *at any time and in any space*, offering a safety net for children whether they're done in the classroom to feel reenergised, in the playground to focus the overstimulated mind or at home as part of a bedtime routine. In this chapter there are several activities to choose from that will inspire children to experience the benefits of connecting with the breath.

Before participating in any of the mindful breathing activities, consult a medical professional for advice if children or adults experience health concerns, particularly of a respiratory or cardio-vascular nature, or for clarification on the suitability of any breathing activities. Consideration of specific needs, personal safety and emotional well-being are paramount, so please be mindful at all times. The mindful breathing activities are for guidance purposes only and do not act as a replacement for medical treatment.

BREATHE

Learn how to breathe mindfully with these simple, diaphragmatic breathing techniques.

Notice the Breath

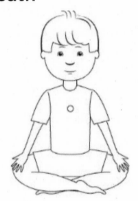

Many children are unaware that breathing is keeping them alive. Slowing down to consciously notice every inhale and exhale can be a peaceful experience.

1. Sit in a comfortable position with the shoulders down and feet flat on the ground.

2. Breathe naturally through the nose for 30 seconds.

3. Notice any sensations in the body.

4. After 30 seconds, begin to experiment by taking in longer inhales and exhales.

5. Continue breathing deeply and equally through the nose for another 30 seconds.

6. Notice any sensations in the body and how the mind feels.

7. Return to breathing naturally.

Once the children have practised noticing the breath and can feel the calming effects, vary the timing so the exhale is longer than the inhale, and experiment further by asking the children to inhale through the nose and exhale through the mouth.

Therapeutic Benefits

- Calming and invigorating
- Improves focus and concentration
- Relieves tension and stress from the body and mind

Developmental Skills

- Body awareness
- Self-care and organisation
- Planning and sequencing

Be Mindful

If required, simplify this activity further by asking the children to breathe deeply for a short while and notice how it feels. Visuals can be presented to prompt the children when they should mindfully breathe in and when they should breathe out, with the visuals being phased out gradually to encourage the children to consciously breathe independently. Alternatively, for more able children, additional instructions can be given to breathe in calm, positive energy and breathe out unwanted feelings and stale energy. If required, use a visual timer to help the children understand the duration of 30 seconds.

Belly Breathing

You will need...

- Sensory Toys

Abdominal or Belly Breathing gives children the kinaesthetic benefit of feeling the effect of the breath on the body with their hands or an object, which can be incredibly calming.

1. Lie down on a comfortable flat surface with the back and legs straight.

2. Place one hand on the chest and the other hand on the belly.

3. Close the eyes.

4. Slowly and mindfully breathe in and out through the nose.

5. Notice the belly fill up with air as it moves up and come down when the air is released. The chest moves very gently each time.

6. Feel the sensations of the hands moving in sync with the breathing.

7. After three minutes of breathing steadily, place a sensory soft toy on the belly.

8. Gently rest both hands on the sensory toy.

9. Continue to breathe mindfully whilst the toy moves up and down on the belly for as long as required.

Teddy bears and other light objects can be placed on the belly if small sensory toys are not available. Once children become confident with this activity and feel calm, control the breath by breathing quickly for a few seconds to notice how the toy moves up and down or falls off the stomach.

Therapeutic Benefits

- Improves focus and attention skills
- Relaxes the whole body and mind
- Has a grounding effect on the body
- Enhances play and social skills
- Stimulates the senses

Developmental Skills

- Body awareness
- Fine motor
- Crosses the midline
- Cognitive learning
- Planning and sequencing

Be Mindful

If required, provide hand-over-hand support to help the children put their hands on the toy or the body for periods of time. Encourage the children to consciously breathe throughout the activity and to notice how objects can move on the body because they are breathing.

Counting the Breath

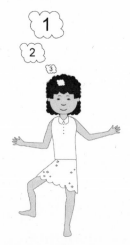

You will need...

- Optional: numerical visuals and objects to represent numbers (e.g. number cards, digital timer or analogue clock)

When children bring their attention towards the logical concept of counting numbers, the mind naturally begins to slow down, and anxious feelings start to ease. There are several methods of counting with the breath. In each counting-the-breath activity below, remind the children to count to themselves silently and, if required, show them visual number prompts.

Count each breath

1. Breathe in deeply – count one.

2. Breathe out – count two.

3. Breathe in – count three.

4. Breathe out – count four.

5. Continue to breathe mindfully up to the count of ten. Alternatively, count up to 20, or as far as it is necessary (depending on the children's cognitive ability) to calm the children down.

Breathing to 4-4-4

1. Breathe in deeply for the count of four.

2. Retain the breath for the count of four.

3. Exhale fully and slowly to the count of four.

4. Continue for four more breathing rounds.

If the children are unable to retain the breath with the count to four, simply focus on inhaling and exhaling to the count of four each time.

Breathing to 7-11

1. Breathe in deeply for the count of seven.

2. Breathe out for the count of 11.

3. Continue for five more breathing rounds.

If the children find it difficult to breathe in and out to the pace of 7-11, adapt the count to shorter intervals to ensure they feel comfortable.

Therapeutic Benefits

- Calms, refocuses and slows down the mind
- Distracts the mind and brings the attention inwards
- Improves concentration and thinking skills
- Helps release pent-up emotions

Developmental Skills

- Cognitive learning
- Self-care and organisation
- Planning and sequencing

Be Mindful

Show numerical visuals and count along with the children who are unable to count or recognise the concept of numbers. Physical props can be used to match the amount of numbers if this does not cause a distraction. Adapt any of the activities above to suit the children's level of understanding.

Advanced Breathing Technique: Alternate Breath (Nadi Shodhan or Anuloma Viloma Pranayama)

Only introduce Alternate Breath to children who have practised other simple mindful-breathing activities and are aware of why this concept is used.

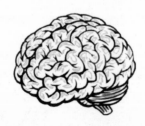

Alternate Breath is an ancient breathing technique used to restore imbalances in the brain and calm the nervous system. The inhale and exhale of the breath alternates between nostrils. The left nostril calms the feeling sensations within the mind and body, whilst the right nostril boosts logic and energetic flow.

1. Sit in a comfortable position with the back straight.

2. Cover the right nostril with the thumb on the right hand.

3. Breathe in slowly through the left nostril.

4. Pause for a moment.

5. Cover the left nostril with the fourth finger of the right hand and release the thumb off the right nostril.

6. Breathe out slowly through the right nostril.

7. Breathe in through the right nostril.

8. Pause for a moment.

9. Cover the right nostril with the thumb and release the fourth finger off the left nostril.

10. Breathe out through the left nostril.

11. Continue for three more rounds or for as long as necessary.

Where necessary, simplify the instructions above to suit the children's level of understanding. The level of detail in the instructions and the process of connecting the breath to movements of the fourth finger and thumb (Surya Ravi Mudra) mean that Alternate Breath may be suited to older children and teenagers. Traditionally, yogis use the fourth finger to enhance the healing benefits of this breathing activity. However, for a simplified version of Alternate Breath or a way to gradually work towards the full activity, start by using the index fingers of both hands to cover the nostrils in turn and then breathe slowly through each nostril.

Therapeutic Benefits

- Calms the mind and increases mental clarity
- Improves concentration and thinking skills
- Revitalises the body and enhances relaxation
- Restores imbalances in the brain
- Calms the emotional state
- Improves hand–eye coordination
- Stimulates the senses, particularly tactile and olfactory ones

Developmental Skills

- Body awareness
- Fine motor
- Visual perception
- Cognitive learning
- Crosses the midline
- Self-care and organisation
- Planning and sequencing

Be Mindful

To support children to understand the planning and sequencing of this breathing activity, provide visuals with prompts about which finger to use each time and indicate the nostril to breathe in and out of. For children with fine motor difficulties, provide hand-over-hand support using the index fingers from both hands to breathe in turn. With more able children who have practised this activity several times, introduce a count to four or five with every inhale and exhale.

SENSORY

Let go of the busy mind and use these breathing activities to stimulate and regulate the senses. For a detailed explanation on the sensory systems see Sensory Yoga on page 109.

Blowing Bubbles

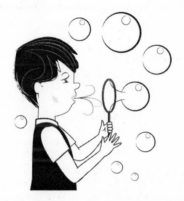

You will need...

- Bottle of bubbles

The simple act of blowing bubbles can tap into children's visual (see), tactile (touch), gustatory (taste), auditory (hear) and interoception (inner sensations) senses whilst enhancing a pleasurable state of focus and calm.

1. Stand or sit in a comfortable position.

2. Hold the bottle of bubbles in one hand.

3. Take a deep breath in for the count of four through the nostrils.

4. Plunge the dipper into the bubble mix with the other hand.

5. Remove the dipper from the bottle and blow bubbles with a long exhale through the mouth to the count of six or for as long as possible.

Continue blowing bubbles for as long as required, either for fun or to calm children down. When the children are well versed in blowing bubbles, mindfully watch the bubbles float and carefully listen to the popping sound. To avoid overstimulation, set clear boundaries by pausing in between each breathing round to observe the bubbles floating and popping. In addition, use an egg timer to remind the children how much time they have to blow bubbles and mindfully inform them of the remaining time towards the end of the session.

Therapeutic Benefits

- Calming and invigorating

- Improves focus and concentration

- Enhances play and social skills

- Strengthens hand–eye coordination

- Stimulates the senses

Developmental Skills

- Fine motor

- Oral motor

- Visual perception and tracking

- Planning and sequencing

Be Mindful

Provide hand-over-hand support for children with fine motor difficulties. For children who are unable to blow bubbles independently, adult assistance or bubble machines can be used as an alternative. To develop cognition and a greater sense of calm, include the Mind Bubbles visualisation from Section 6: Visualisation on page 83.

Travelling Objects

You will need...

- Light sensory props or objects to blow on (examples include scarves, cotton wool, feathers, rice, pom-poms)
- Straws to blow through

Observing objects as they travel with the breath creates a visual for children to see first-hand the power of breathing mindfully. Scarves, cotton wool, feathers, rice, ping pong balls, short pieces of string, pom-poms and other light objects can be used as sensory props for this activity.

1. Sit or stand in a comfortable position.

2. Place a small handful of objects in one hand.

3. Take a deep breath in through the nose to the count of five.

4. Blow on the objects with a long exhale through the mouth until the hand is empty.

5. Change hands to repeat this activity.

Travelling Objects can also be completed on a flat surface with the children blowing the objects from one place to another, e.g. towards the end of the yoga mat or towards a visual target on a table.

Therapeutic Benefits

- Alerts the mind to become present
- Improves focus and concentration
- Enhances play and social skills
- Strengthens hand–eye coordination
- Stimulates the senses

Developmental Skills

- Oral motor

- Fine motor

- Visual perception and tracking

- Planning and sequencing

Be Mindful

If some children require additional support with oral motor skills, adults and other children can help blow the light objects on their behalf or use a handheld fan. If some children have fine motor difficulties or require support to hold their hand in position, adults can gently rest the children's hands on top of theirs and then provide hand-over-hand support to pick up any objects. More able children can use straws to blow through and move the light objects. Alternatively, they can partner up with other children to blow the light objects back and forth between them.

Squidgy Sensory Toys

You will need...

- Squidgy fidget toys (examples include Wibbly Worms, Squidgy Teddies and stress balls)

The calming and highly tactile benefits of soft, squeezable sensory toys encourage children to explore and engage in the senses. Made from flexible textures and materials, squidgy sensory toys, also known as fidget toys, entice children to experiment with touch and develop early play skills.

1. Place the squidgy toy in the palms of both hands.

2. Take a deep breath in through the nose whilst cupping the hands to squeeze the squidgy toy.

3. Exhale through the mouth as the hands gently release and still hold the squidgy toy.

4. Continue for four more breathing rounds or as long as necessary.

For comfort, and as an alternative to using both hands, children can squeeze the squidgy toy with one hand each time while following the breathing routine above.

Therapeutic Benefits

- Provides a soothing tactile distraction
- Boosts focus, concentration and attention skills
- Enhances play and social skills
- Stimulates the senses
- Improves hand–eye coordination

Developmental Skills

- Body awareness
- Fine motor
- Cognitive learning
- Self-care and organisation
- Planning and sequencing

Be Mindful

The children may need lots of verbal or visual prompts to coordinate and sync the inhale and exhale breaths with the movement of the hands. Remind the children to notice the sensations of the belly inflating and deflating. If appropriate, after the children have practised a few rounds, the adults can place their hands gently on the children's shoulders to help them keep the shoulders down. Provide hand-over-hand support for children with fine motor or tactile difficulties. Give clear boundaries if required, and set visual timers if it is likely that children will become overstimulated whilst using squidgy toys.

Blow Ball Pipe

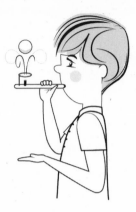

You will need...

- Blow ball pipe
- Light polystyrene ball
- Optional: pom-poms, cotton wool, large feathers and other light objects

Blowing through the ball pipe can be a fun and creative way for children to improve their focus and concentration and strengthen their connection to the breath.

1. Place the lips around the suction end of the pipe.

2. The ball rests gently at the open end of the pipe.

3. Take a deep breath through the nose and puff the cheeks.

4. Blow with an extended exhale through the mouth to lift the ball up.

5. Continue to inhale and exhale for three more rounds to try to make the ball hover for as long as possible.

To make this activity achievable for children, use polystyrene balls, large pom-poms or other light objects that require reduced amounts of air to keep the object floating above the pipe.

For added sensory awareness and visual pleasure, vary the colours and shapes of the light objects blown upon.

Therapeutic Benefits

- Alerts the mind and energy towards a focal point

- Improves focus and concentration

- Enhances play and social skills

- Stimulates the senses

Developmental Skills

- Fine motor

- Oral motor

- Visual perception and tracking

- Planning and sequencing

Be Mindful

Do not do this activity if children are very young or have respiratory problems or oral motor difficulties due to the likelihood of them attempting to swallow small objects and the intensity of the exhales through the mouth to keep the ball up. Ensure children are supervised and *do not* exhale for too long each time, as this may cause lightheaded dizziness. Provide hand-over-hand support to position and hold the stem of the pipe for any children with fine motor difficulties. If required, use visual prompts to show the target height for the ball.

Parachute

You will need...

- Play parachute

With a small group of children, the effect of raising the parachute up into the air and then lowering the material to float back down can be incredibly fun, particularly during playful activities connected to the breath. In this activity the children pretend to be turtles popping into their shell to relax. The parachute represents the turtle's shell.

1. Stand in a circle with each child holding on to the handles around the edge of the parachute.

2. Instruct the children to raise the parachute.

3. As the parachute is lifted by the group, the adult slowly counts to three.

4. The group takes a deep breath in sync with the adult's count to three.

5. Lower the parachute to another count of three as the group exhales.

6. Repeat this for three rounds to settle the group into the rhythm of conscious breathing.

7. Inform the group that it's time for the turtles to rest under the shell.

8. Choose one child to sit underneath the parachute (turtle shell).

9. The rest of the group slowly counts to three and lifts the parachute whilst the child underneath the parachute takes in a deep breath in sync with the count of three.

10. The group counts to three again, as the parachute is lowered and the child underneath the parachute exhales.

11. Repeat the breathing activity with the same child for two more rounds.

12. After the third round, the child crawls out from under the shell.

13. Take turns so every child in the group has a turn under the parachute.

If a parachute is not available use soft, stretchy material or a large blanket as an alternative.

Therapeutic Benefits

- Directs attention towards a focal point
- Boosts and alerts energy levels
- Encourages cooperation and turn-taking
- Enhances play and social skills
- Stimulates the senses
- Improves hand–eye coordination

Developmental Skills

- Body awareness
- Gross motor
- Fine motor
- Oral motor and phonological awareness
- Cognitive learning
- Planning and sequencing

Be Mindful

If the children become excitable during parachute games, give lots of calm and clear adult prompts to set firm boundaries beforehand and to ensure everyone in the group is aware of the expectations. Provide full support, modelling and verbal prompts for children experiencing difficulties when following instructions and/or holding the parachute.

Mirror Fogging

You will need...

- Mirror or suitable reflective object

Mirrors are reflective sensory tools that give children visual feedback as they explore self-image, contrast shades of light and develop play skills. Mirror Fogging, or invisible breath as it is sometimes known, is a fun and relaxing way for children to see their breath come to life.

1. Look closely at your own eyes using a mirror.
2. Breathe in and out deeply for ten seconds.
3. Inhale through the nose for the count of four.
4. Breathe out through the mouth onto the mirror for the count of six.
5. Observe how the mirror fogs up.
6. Continue for three more rounds.
7. Remember to listen carefully to the breath on every exhale.

As an alternative, windows and other reflective materials can be used for this breathing activity, particularly during long car or train journeys. Encourage all the children to mindfully explore their self-image in the mirror as they see themselves breathe in and out, particularly if they experience difficulties using the breath to fog up the mirror.

Therapeutic Benefits

- Provides a calming visual and auditory distraction
- Improves concentration and attention skills
- Enhances creative play and social skills
- Stimulates the senses

Developmental Skills

- Body awareness

- Oral motor and phonological awareness

- Cognitive learning

- Visual perception

- Self-care and organisation

Be Mindful

Ensure the mirrors used are suitable to the age group and skills of the children using them. For younger children, it may be more appropriate to use plastic reflective materials. If any children have oral motor difficulties or require additional support, adults can breathe on the mirror with the children or on their behalf, whilst the children participate by looking at their reflections as they breathe in and out. More able children can cup their hands around their mouths to help contain and focus the breath towards the mirror and then use the fingers to make shapes in the condensation.

Expanding Ball

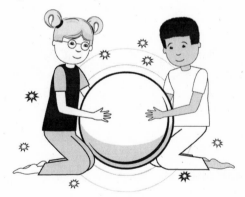

You will need...

- Hoberman sphere
- Visual/verbal prompts to open and close the ball using the breath

The Hoberman sphere, also known as the Expanding Ball, was created by Chuck Hoberman, an inventor of folding toys and structures. The repetitive motion of the sphere folding inwards and outwards can be used as a breathing tool to help children connect to the breath.

1. Sit or stand in a comfortable position with the spine straight.

2. Inform the children they will be breathing in sync with the actions of the ball.

3. Ensure the ball is closed at the start of this activity.

4. Slowly open the expanding ball and ask the children to breathe in deeply through the nose.

5. Gradually close the ball as the children exhale slowly through the mouth (or nose) with the action of the ball.

6. Continue breathing deeply and mindfully along with the ball for five more rounds.

Aim for the opening and closing of the ball (inhale and exhale motion) to be the same amount of time but adapt this to a longer exhale if children are experiencing heightened emotions. When children become more aware of Expanding Ball breathing, give the ball to them to gain the kinaesthetic experience of the hand and breathing motion.

Therapeutic Benefits

- Calms and soothes the mind
- Improves focus and concentration
- Enhances play and social skills

- Strengthens hand–eye coordination
- Stimulates the senses

Developmental Skills

- Fine motor
- Visual perception
- Cognitive learning
- Planning and sequencing
- Self-care and organisation

Be Mindful

Provide hand-over-hand support for children with fine motor and visual processing difficulties. With more able children, add additional verbal reminders by asking them to observe how their belly fills up like a balloon with fresh cleansing oxygen and then deflates to release negative thoughts and feelings whenever they exhale. For added sensory pleasure, use a 'glow in the dark' Hoberman sphere with soft lighting to soothe the senses.

Sensory Cuddle Swing

You will need...

- Therapy swing hammock
- Hanging equipment

A swinging motion with a cuddling sensation on the whole body can help self-regulate overstimulated children and enhance a calmer state. Hammocks are often used as sensory swings for children on the autistic spectrum and those with sensory processing disorder. Sensory swings are made of stretchy material to recreate the human touch and often come in warm colours to calm the mind and stimulate creativity.

1. Have the children lay comfortably in the sensory swing.

2. Ask the children when they are ready for the swing to move.

3. Gently move the swing to sway from left to right.

4. Give the children time to swing gently until they become calm.

5. If appropriate, gradually introduce the idea of connecting the breath to the motion of the swing, e.g. breathe in when the swing moves to the left and breathe out when the swing moves to the right.

Blankets and other large materials can be used if a sensory swing is not available. If children are calm and settled but want to stay in the sensory swing, provide a visual timer to let them known how much time they have remaining.

Therapeutic Benefits

- Provides calm for the whole body and mind

- Improves focus and draws the attention inwards

- Soothes heightened emotions

- Stimulates the senses, particularly the vestibular system

Developmental Skills

- Body awareness

- Gross motor

- Planning and sequencing

- Self-care and organisation

Be Mindful

For safety and comfort, ensure the hammock is securely fastened at both ends. If the hammock is handheld, check the adults are holding it at the same height from both ends. If the children are unable to connect with the breath during the sensory swing, adults can model this (provided it does not create too much of a distraction) by breathing in audibly as the swing moves to one side and then breathing out as the swing moves to the other side. Encourage the children to communicate either verbally or with visuals how they would like the swing to sway. In many cases, children enjoy listening to calming music during the sensory swing, so present this as an option once children become comfortable with the process.

ANIMAL BREATHING

Ignite children's imagination and join the animal kingdom with these creative breathing exercises.

Lion's Breath (Simhasana Pranayama)

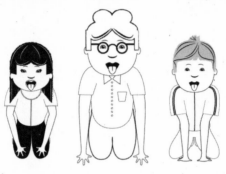

Lion's Breath is an ancient yoga breathing technique to release pent up-energy, including stress, anxiety and anger, from the upper body. Ask children to imagine they are powerful, brave lions getting ready to make almighty roars.

1. Sit on the heels with the hands rested on the knees or on the floor.

2. Take in a big inhale through the nose.

3. Tilt the body forward with the jaw stretched open and stick the tongue out.

4. Exhale through the mouth for as long as possible whilst letting out a big, loud 'ROARRRRR' during the exhale!

In traditional yoga circles, the 'HA' sound is used rather than the roar, which is used to get children into the lion character, so choose the most suitable sound and repeat this activity for three to four rounds.

Therapeutic Benefits

- Relieves tension in the upper body and alerts the mind
- Increases blood circulation to the face
- Improves self-esteem and confidence
- Calming and invigorating

Developmental Skills

- Body awareness
- Gross motor
- Fine motor
- Oral motor and phonological awareness
- Auditory discrimination
- Self-care and organisation

Be Mindful

To support non-verbal children, the adult can make the 'roar' or 'HA' sound on their behalf, or the children can pretend to be lions that roar quietly. For children with poor fine or gross motor skills, provide hands-on support with the posture (straight back leaning forward) and check the amount of pressure the child is placing on the hands as the body leans forward.

Bunny Breath

Bunnies are very alert little animals because they regularly sniff in short bursts of air. Bunny Breathing is a cleansing and awakening activity to help children focus. This activity is often used to support symptoms of ADHD. Inform the children that they are little bunnies wriggling their noses and sniffing the air for carrots.

1. Sit on the shins with the back straight and chest lifted.

2. Tuck in the chin and breathe in for three quick, short inhales (sniffs) through the nostrils.

3. Make a long exhale (sigh) through the nose.

Repeat the breathing activity for five to seven rounds.

Therapeutic Benefits

*   Cleanses, relaxes and alerts the mind and body

*   Awakens and focuses the brain

*   Boosts energy levels

*   Stimulates the senses

Developmental Skills

*   Body awareness

*   Self-care and organisation

*   Planning and sequencing

Be Mindful

For children who are unable to sit on their shins, standing or seated positions can be used as alternatives. For added fun, ask the children to hop around as bunnies and/or place their hands on the sides of their heads to create bunny ears. If the children begin to feel dizzy, they should pause to breathe normally and then, if appropriate, restart the activity or move on to a more suitable breathing activity.

Fish Breath

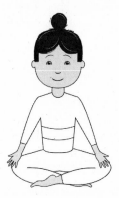

Fish Breath is a soothing and fun breathing activity to help children during bouts of anxiety. Gradually releasing the breath using sound refocuses the mind and slows down the body.

1. Take a big, deep breath in through the nose to fill the belly and chest.

2. Expand and puff the cheeks like a fish with the mouth closed.

3. Slowly exhale using short, quick bursts through the mouth, making 'bloop' sounds to mimic a fish each time.

Repeat three or four times or for as long as necessary.

Therapeutic Benefits

- Reenergises and calms the mind and body
- Build's self-esteem
- Increases lung capacity
- Enhances play and social skills

Developmental Skills

- Oral motor and phonological awareness
- Body awareness
- Self-care and organisation
- Auditory discrimination

Be Mindful

If children have oral motor difficulties, avoid puffing the cheeks to make the 'bloop' sound. Instead, focus on gently opening and closing the mouth to exhale. Please consult a medical practitioner before this activity to check the suitability for children with respiratory ailments.

Whale Breath

Whales often glide through the water with great ease and flow, and then, all of a sudden, excess water gushes through the blowhole in full force. Whale Breath is a fun and creative breathing activity that is ideal to help children with anger issues.

1. Sit with the back straight, chin tucked in and shoulders down.

2. Place the wrists together with the palms and fingers open to create a cup shape with the hands.

3. Raise the arms to put the cupped hands on the crown of the head. This is the whale's blowhole.

4. Tilt the head up.

5. Breathe in through the nostrils and puff up the cheeks.

6. Pause with the breath for the count of five with the cupped hands still on the head.

7. With a vibrant exhale, create an explosion sound from the mouth. At the same time, shoot the hands and arms quickly up, out to the sides and back down towards the knees.

Aim to create a dramatic effect with the arms during the exhale. Inform the children that the blowhole has just released all the unwanted thoughts and feelings. Repeat for four rounds or for as long as necessary.

Therapeutic Benefits

- Relieves tension from the face, neck, shoulders and upper back
- Releases negative emotions
- Calms and refocuses the mind
- Improves hand–eye coordination
- Builds core strength

Developmental Skills

- Body awareness
- Oral motor and phonological awareness
- Gross motor
- Fine motor
- Auditory discrimination

Be Mindful

For children who are physically unable to move their hands and arms, provide hand-over-hand support or simply focus on breathing in deeply and exaggerate the exhale to create the explosion sound. For children who experience oral motor difficulties, create the explosion sound on their behalf and adapt the activity for their level of ability.

Bee Breath (Bhramari Pranayama)

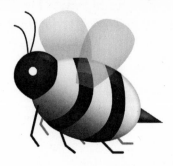

Named after a black Indian humming bee, Bhramari or Bee Breath calms and focuses the mind. Often used with children who have ADHD, anxiety and obsessive compulsive disorder (OCD), Bee Breath directs the children's attention inwards.

1. Sit in a comfortable position with the back straight, chest open and eyes closed or gently gazing down.

2. Place the thumbs firmly over each ear flap (pinna) to prevent hearing.

3. With the thumbs still firmly covering the ear flaps, raise both elbows just above the shoulders and rest the little fingers of both hands where the hairline meets the forehead.

4. Place the rest of the fingers on the crown of the head pointing towards each other. The hands now create a helmet over the head (Shanmukhi Mudra).

5. Take a long, deep inhale through the nose and breathe out through the nose to make a long humming sound.

Repeat for four rounds, or for as long as necessary. The vibration of the humming can help harmonise inner turmoil and relieve tension. Yogis can also spread and lay the fingers across the face with the thumbs over the ear flaps to feel the vibration across their face. Children can benefit from placing one hand on the chest and the other on their stomach to feel and experience the bodily sensations of the humming.

Therapeutic Benefits

- Calms the mind and body
- Soothes physical, mental and emotional well-being
- Encourages relaxation
- Decreases blood pressure
- Improves sleep

Developmental Skills

- Body awareness
- Gross motor
- Fine motor
- Oral motor and phonological awareness
- Stimulates the senses
- Self-care and organisation
- Auditory discrimination

Be Mindful

For children with poor fine motor skills, make humming sounds without the Shanmukhi Mudra. To support non-verbal children, adults can make the 'hum' sound on their behalf or use a musical instrument with a low tone.

Elephant Breath

Named after the largest land animal, the Elephant Breath can energise and wake children up if they feel tired or are experiencing low emotions. Elephant Breath is a fun and strengthening, whole-body activity for children.

1. Stand with the feet wide apart and back straight.

2. Interlace the fingers, bend the knees slightly and dangle the arms between the legs to make an elephant trunk.

3. Breathe in and out deeply three times whilst dangling the arms between the legs with the head facing downwards in ragdoll yoga pose (Uttanasana).

4. Take a big inhale through the nose whilst raising the arms (trunk), with the fingers still interlaced, high above the head.

5. Lean back very gently for a 'quick shower' from the trunk.

6. Exhale through the mouth whilst swinging the arms back down through the legs swiftly and make the noise of an elephant.

7. After three rounds, stay standing upright with the arms above the head (trunk). Safely arch the back to be showered with kindness, peaceful energy and strength.

Therapeutic Benefits

- Invigorates the mind and body
- Increases confidence
- Relieves tension from the shoulders
- Stretches the legs and back
- Improves hand–eye coordination

Developmental Skills

- Body awareness
- Gross motor
- Fine motor
- Crosses the midline
- Planning and sequencing
- Auditory discrimination

Be Mindful

Gross and fine motor hand-over-hand support may be required to help children maintain a standing position, cross the midline and interlace their fingers. Alternatively, children can be seated in a chair if they are unable to stand for lengths of time or experience problems with the spine. Invite more able children to choose anything that makes them feel happy and calm to shower themselves with.

Dog Breath

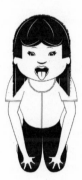

Panting like a dog can be fun and detoxifying for children. Dog Breath increases the oxygen intake to the brain and can help settle emotions. Sit or stand in a comfortable position with the back straight and chest open. Inform the children that dogs pant to cool down, and this brings lots of calming energy into and around into their bodies.

1.   Take in a deep breath through the nostrils.

2.   Open the mouth with the tongue stretched out and gently resting on the bottom lip.

3.   Pant through the mouth like an excited dog for 30 seconds.

4.   Close the mouth to breathe in and out deeply through the nose for 15 seconds.

5.   Open the mouth again with the tongue out and pant like a dog.

Do this activity for two to three rounds. Remember to pause and breathe deeply in between rounds.

Therapeutic Benefits

- Cleanses, detoxifies and alerts the mind and body

- Strengthens and tones abdominal muscles

- Releases negative emotions

- Increases energy levels

- Stimulates the senses

Developmental Skills

- Body awareness

- Oral motor and phonological awareness

- Gross motor (core muscles)

Be Mindful

If children require support with oral motor skills, ask them to keep the tongue in the mouth whilst panting and ensure the mouth is relaxed. For added fun, with children who have a strong core and are able to balance on their hands and knees, maintain the 'table top' position during the panting. Please consult a medical professional or trained yoga instructor *before* practising Dog Breath on children with epilepsy, asthma and abdominal difficulties. Pregnant adults should also receive guidance before practising this activity.

Bear Breath

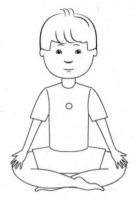

Named after one of the largest animals, Bear Breath symbolises the peace and rest that bears experience during hibernation. This is a calming activity to bring children into a peaceful and grounded state.

1. Sit in a chair or on the floor crossed legged. Ensure the back is straight, shoulders are down and chest is open.

2. Close the eyes and breathe through the nostrils to the count of five.

3. Pause with the breath for the count of three.

4. Breathe out through the nose for a count of five.

5. Pause for the count of three.

Continue for five rounds or as long as necessary. For similar counting-the-breath activities, see Counting the Breath on page 28.

Therapeutic Benefits

- Enhances a sense of peace and mental clarity

- Refocuses the mind

- Releases negative emotions

- Increases lung capacity

Developmental Skills

- Body awareness

- Cognitive learning

- Planning and sequencing

- Self-care and organisation

Be Mindful

For children who experience difficulties with planning, sequencing and counting numbers, provide visual pictorial support, a timer and/or verbal prompts. Pausing with the breath for a count of three and inhaling each time to the count of five may take some practice and understanding, so patience, lots of repetition and adult modelling during the process may be required.

Snake Breath

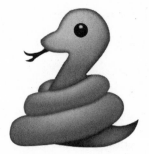

Snake Breath brings children into the slow, smooth and meditative state of the snake. This is ideal for children experiencing heightened emotions, because the hissing sound of a snake can give a soothing sensation of releasing air.

1. Sit or stand in a comfortable position.

2. Breathe in through the nose for as long as possible.

3. Notice the belly inflating.

4. Steadily make the loud hissing sound of a snake whilst slowly exhaling through the mouth.

5. Ensure all of the air from the stomach is gradually released and the shoulders are relaxed.

6. Take another deep breath in to start again.

Repeat for three to five rounds.

Therapeutic Benefits

- Develops focus and calms the mind

- Releases tension from the body

- Helps prevent oral diseases

- Increases lung capacity

Developmental Skills

- Body awareness

- Oral motor and phonological awareness

- Auditory discrimination

- Planning and sequencing

Be Mindful

For non-verbal children with oral motor difficulties, create the hissing sound on their behalf whilst they learn to breathe in deeply through the nose and exhale slowly through the mouth. If the children are physically able, after practising for three or four rounds suggest they do the cobra or snake pose (Bhujangasana) whilst they make the hissing sound.

SHAPE BREATHING

Focus on the breath whilst engaging both hemispheres of the brain with shape breathing.

Star Breathing

You will need...

- Visual of a star

Breathing around a visual of a five-point star and counting the breath is a creative and aspirational way to help children feel focused and calm.

1. Before you start, lay a copy of the visual of a large star on a flat surface for each child, and ensure the children are in a comfortable seated position.

2. Place the index finger of the dominant hand at the bottom left point of the star.

3. Slowly breathe in whilst the finger moves diagonally up, tracing the outline of the star.

4. Pause at the first inner corner of the star, retaining the breath for five seconds.

5. Breathe out as the finger moves towards the next point of the star.

6. You are now at the middle left corner of the star –
    breathe in whilst moving the finger along to the next
    inner corner.

7. Pause at this corner for five seconds.

8. Continue breathing in and out around the star
    remembering to pause for five seconds at every inner
    corner.

9. Change direction and breathe around the star from right
    to left.

Once the children are well versed in breathing around the star,
to add a variety give them a choice of other shapes to breathe
around, e.g. a square, triangle or hexagon or around the outline
of objects.

Therapeutic Benefits

- Calms and focuses the mind

- Relieves stress

- Improves hand–eye coordination

- Enhances creative play skills

Developmental Skills

- Visual perception and tracking

- Fine motor

- Cognitive learning

- Planning and sequencing

Be Mindful

If children are unable to visually track and trace their finger around
the star, provide additional verbal prompts and hand-over-hand
support, particularly if they experience fine motor difficulties. Ask
more able children to visualise the star in the night sky and use

their index finger to breathe around an imaginary star floating in front of them.

Bubble (Circle) Reading

You will need...

- Bubble (Circle) Reading sheet from Section 2 of Part V: Resources

Bubble Reading is a way to read a picture book containing rows of bubbles. Children mindfully breathe in sync when tracking large and small bubbles from left to right. Bubble Reading gradually makes children feel focused and more at ease.

1. Place a sheet of paper (see Section 2 of Part V: Resources) with rows of large and small circles in front of the children. These circles are breathing bubbles: ○∘∘○○∘○○○∘∘

2. Use the index finger to point at the first bubble on the top left of the page and breathe in and out through the nose according to the size of the bubble:

   - large bubble: take a deep breath in and out

   - small bubble: take a shallow breath in and out.

3. Continue breathing and moving the finger slowly along each row of bubbles from left to right and down the page.

In Bubble Reading, the large bubbles should always outnumber the small bubbles on each row to ensure children experience the calming benefits of breathing deeply. See Section 2 of Part V: Resources for an example of a Bubble Reading activity.

Therapeutic Benefits

- Focuses the mind and body

- Develops concentration

- Improves hand–eye coordination

- Brings the attention directly into the present

Developmental Skills

- Fine motor

- Visual perception and tracking

- Cognitive learning

- Planning and sequencing

Be Mindful

Ensure the amount of bubbles per row is consistent with children's needs and abilities, as too many breathing bubbles on a sheet of paper may, in some cases, cause overstimulation. Remind children to breathe along each row slowly and mindfully. Provide hand-over-hand support and verbal prompts for children with fine motor and visual tracking difficulties. For added fun and visual impact with more able children, ask them to draw their own bubbles and colour each bubble in with their favourite colours.

Take 5 Breathing

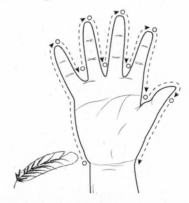

You will need...

- Soft objects to trace around hand/fingers (e.g. feathers, pom-poms)

Also known as Finger Breathing, Take 5 Breathing is a relaxing way for children to spread their fingers and create a star shape and then focus on the breath whilst tracing the finger and physically connecting with themselves in the present moment.

1. Open one hand (with the palm facing you) in front of the face at eye level.

2. Place the index finger of the other hand on the wrist.

3. Breathe in through the nose as the index finger gently traces the side of the first finger/thumb on the left towards the fingertip.

4. Breathe out through the nose as the index finger moves down the inside of the first finger/thumb.

5. Continue tracing the outline of the hand and breathe in every time the index finger traces upwards towards the fingertips and breathe out every time it moves down.

6. When the index finger reaches the right side of the wrist, pause for five seconds.

7. Breathe in as the index finger moves back up the last finger/thumb on the right.

8. Continue to breathe around the hand until the index finger is back on the left side of the wrist.

9. Change hands to do this on the other hand.

Young children or anyone sensitive to touch may prefer the sensation of using feathers, pom-poms or other soft objects to trace around each finger. After practising Take 5 for a few rounds, invite the children to experiment by exhaling through the mouth each time and notice how this feels.

Therapeutic Benefits

- Calms the mind and enhances mental clarity

- Grounds and connects the mind with the body

- Improves concentration and hand–eye coordination

- Stimulates the senses

Developmental Skills

- Body awareness

- Fine motor

- Oral motor

- Visual perception and tracking

- Crosses the midline

- Planning and sequencing

Be Mindful

Provide hand-over-hand support and verbal prompts for children who experience difficulties with fine motor skills, visual tracking or crossing the midline. Ask physically able children to partner up with another child or adult to breathe and trace around each other's hands. Create printed visuals of handprints to place on a flat surface for children to trace around if they are highly sensitive or unable to physically position their own hands at eye level.

Lazy Eight Breathing

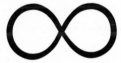

You will need...

- Large visual of infinity symbol

Lazy Eight Breathing is often used to engage the brain and gain mental clarity. Children trace around a horizontal number eight, known as the infinity symbol, and gradually settle into the continued and peaceful flowing motion.

1. Inform the children that Mr Eight is feeling lazy so he's lying down to have a snooze.

2. Point the index finger and place it in the centre of the number to tickle and wake up Mr Eight whilst he's sleeping.

3. Breathe in whilst tracing the finger slowly around the number to the left side in a full loop.

4. Come back to middle of the number and pause for a moment.

5. Breathe out whilst tracing around to the right side of the number eight.

6. Continue with this breathing action around the figure eight for three rounds. Change the direction of the finger for another three rounds. Repeat as necessary.

Lazy Eight Breathing can be done with printed visuals or with children drawing the number eight horizontally in the air.

Therapeutic Benefits

-   Relaxes and calms the mind and body

-   Develops focus and attention skills

-   Balances emotions

-   Improves hand–eye coordination

Developmental Skills

-   Fine motor

-   Visual perception and tracking

-   Planning and sequencing

-   Crosses the midline

Be Mindful

To remind children when to swap between breathing in and out, a yellow star or dot could be placed at the centre of the lazy eight. Provide hand-over-hand support and verbal prompts for children who experience difficulties with fine motor skills, visual tracking and/or crossing the midline.

SOUND

Explore and create sound vibrations and then feel the calming sensations.

Ocean Breath (Ujjayi Pranayama)

You will need...

- Mirror or reflective object

Ocean Breath encourages the constant flow of breath into the body and a peaceful connection to the mind. This breathing activity is particularly great for anxious or depressed children, as it can create the calming and reenergising sensation of being by the ocean.

1. Close the eyes and sit in a comfortable position.

2. Breathe in slowly through the nostrils.

3. Imagine the whole body is being filled up with cleansing air.

4. Open the mouth to breathe out and imagine you are fogging up a mirror with every exhale.

5. Listen carefully to the breath.

6. Continue to breathe in through the nose and breathe out through the mouth, creating the sound that you would make if you were fogging up a mirror, for five more rounds.

7. Pause for a moment to feel the relaxing sensations in the whole body.

8. Close the mouth.

9. Breathe in slowly through the nostrils.

10. Breathe out slowly through the nostrils and keep the mouth closed.

11. With the mouth closed continue to make the sound of fogging up the imaginary mirror with every exhale.

12. Now listen carefully to the breaths, which sound just like waves in the ocean.

13. Mindfully continue Ocean Breath until the children become calm.

Due to the complexity of this breathing activity, it may be best suited to older children and teenagers. To work towards this activity gradually or for a simple 'listen to the breath' alternative, Mirror Fogging found on page 42 is a fun sensory breathing activity.

Therapeutic Benefits

- Calms and relaxes the body

- Brings the mind into a meditative state

- Improves focus and concentration

- Enhances creative thinking skills

- Stimulates the senses

Developmental Skills

- Body awareness

- Oral motor and phonological awareness

- Auditory discrimination

- Cognitive learning

- Self-care and organisation

- Planning and sequencing

Be Mindful

If required, simplify the instructions by using less verbal input and some visual prompts to ensure children understand the instructions. Do not practise this activity with children who experience respiratory or oral motor difficulties. Ocean Breath is best practised when seated in a relaxed position, but if children are unable to remain still for a length of time, connect to the breath with mindful movements in Body Flow on page 87.

ॐ Chanting Mantras

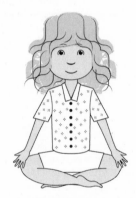

You will need...
• Chanting rhythms or sounds

The chanting of mantras is the simple and effective act of quietening the mind and bringing awareness to the breath through sound. Yoga practitioners believe that chanting the mantra 'Om' creates the sound and vibration of the universe, enabling chanters to deeply connect with inner peace and resonate with the world around them.

1. Close the eyes and sit in a comfortable position.

2. Take in a deep breath through the nose.

3. Open the mouth to exhale and chant 'Om' for as long as the breath will carry the sound. Be sure to pronounce it as: AAAA...UUUUU...MMMMMMMMMMM to create the sound of the chant.

4. Close the mouth to take in a deep breath through the nose.

5. Open the mouth to exhale and chant.

6. Continue chanting with the breath for three or four rounds.

7. Pause to feel the sensations in the body and mind.

8. Keep chanting until the children feel at peace and calm.

If desired, alternative and simple calming phrases or words can be used in place of the Om sound whilst following the steps above. This includes chanting the calming mantra 'Ah' to transform lower energies within the body into creative expression and manifestation.

Mindfully connecting mantras with every inhale and exhale of the breath is often vocalised out loud. However, mantras can also be silently spoken from within the mind:

Silent mantra	Desired effect	Deep breath in through the nose and silently say...	Extended deep breath out through the nose whilst silently saying...
Namaste	Compassion	'Nam'	'aste'
Yoga	Harmony	'Yo'	'ga'
Slow down	Calming	'Slow'	'down'
I'm here	Grounding	'I'm'	'here'
It's okay	Reassuring	'It's'	'okay'
I'm strong	Confidence	'I'm'	'strong'

As shown in the table above, the first syllable or word of the mantra is recited on the inhale and the second part is recited on the long exhale. Adults can direct this process by saying the mantras out loud as children listen and consciously breathe in and out. After lots of practice and adult guidance, more able children can go on to recite mantras in their mind with the breath independently.

Therapeutic Benefits

- Calms the mind and enhances mental clarity
- Reenergises the body and improves concentration
- Releases stress and negative emotions
- Improves self-esteem and self-expression
- Stimulates the senses

Developmental Skills

- Body awareness
- Oral motor and phonological awareness
- Auditory discrimination
- Cognitive learning
- Verbal reasoning
- Self-care and organisation

Be Mindful

Despite the many healing benefits of chanting mantras with children, chanting has, in some cases, been viewed as reciting religious phrasing, so be sure to check you have permission, particularly when chanting the Om sound. If in doubt, sing simple words or phrases out loud that empower, uplift, calm and make children feel good about themselves. Once children are well versed at connecting the breath to the mantra, invite them to place their hands on their chest and/or throat to experience the calming sensation of the sound vibrating through the body. With non-verbal children, practise any of the silent mantras above with the adult chanting out loud or play pre-recorded chanting from an audible device and show children how to consciously breathe along with the sounds they can hear.

Listening to Music

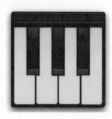

> **You will need...**
>
> - Pre-recorded sounds (e.g. piano, ocean, birds, lullabies, flutes)
> - Musical instruments for live music
> - Audio device

Listening to calm or upbeat music is known to have healing benefits that soothe emotional states, particularly depression and anxiety.

1. Choose a piece of music or sounds related to the children's emotional state:
   - slow music if the children feel stressed or anxious
   - upbeat music if the children feel tired or upset.
2. Play the music out loud or through headphones.
3. Mindfully breathe in and out as the music is being played.
4. Place the hands on the belly to feel the sensation of the breath moving.

The sounds children listen to can be the waves of the ocean, birds chirping, piano, flutes, guitar, lullabies, nature, people marching, audiobooks, meditation music or even children's favourite songs. Encourage independence and creativity by asking children to choose sounds or songs to listen to. If required, provide visuals to represent the different sounds for children to choose from.

Therapeutic Benefits

- Brings the mind into a meditative state

- Improves creativity and thinking skills

- Boosts concentration and stimulates the senses

- Eases muscle tension and relaxes the body

- Enhances emotional regulation

Developmental Skills

- Body awareness

- Cognitive learning

- Auditory discrimination

- Self-care and organisation

- Planning and sequencing

Be Mindful

Where possible, incorporate listening to music into daily routines, particularly during transitions and calming activities. The free-flowing nature of music can be very liberating for children, particularly as music can be listened to anywhere at any time, so be sure to set clear boundaries and show a visual timer if required. If children cover their ears or become overwhelmed, monitor their mood in relation to the pace and tempo of the piece of music, change or stop the sound when required and hold the space where children can freely explore their senses and connect to their creativity.

Playing Musical Instruments

You will need...

- Wind instruments (e.g. horn, flute, harmonica, trumpet)

Playing musical instruments goes hand in hand with mindfulness and instantly brings children's awareness into the here and now. Every musical note created with the breath represents thoughts initially processed in the mind to generate external sound vibrations. These vibrations create internal feelings and sensations within the body and can be fun and incredibly healing for children, as shown in Music Therapy on page 128.

1. Sit or stand in a comfortable position with the back straight and chest open.

2. Choose wind instrument/s to blow through, e.g. whistle, flute, recorder, trumpet, harmonica, party blower or horn.

3. Take a deep breath in.

4. Breathe out with a long exhale to blow and create melodic sound vibrations.

5. Mindfully notice the breath with every inhale and exhale.

6. Continue playing and exploring the instrument at the children's leisure.

In addition, or as an alternative to the wind instrument, children can sing their favourite song or play any other instrument, like the drums, whilst mindfully connecting to the breath.

Therapeutic Benefits

- Calms, focuses and slows down the mind
- Improves creativity and thinking skills
- Enhances emotional regulation
- Relaxes and strengthens the body
- Boosts self-esteem and confidence
- Stimulates all of the senses

Developmental Skills

- Body awareness
- Fine motor
- Oral motor and phonological awareness
- Cognitive learning
- Auditory discrimination
- Visual tracking (if reading music)
- Planning and sequencing

Be Mindful

Remember to have fun with this activity whilst connecting to the breath. There are strong fine and oral motor elements of this breathing activity, so be realistic with expectations and encourage children to choose and play instruments they feel comfortable with. For children who would like to develop their musical skills further, work with a professional music teacher to enhance their creative skills and learn how to read music.

VISUALISATION

Experience the power and creativity of using the imagination.

Imaginary Breath

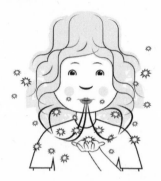

> **You will need...**
>
> - Optional: physical props to support the visualisation activities

Many children enjoy listening to stories and using their imagination to visualise characters, events and settings as the story unfolds. Connecting the breath with the imagination is a simple, fun and creative way for children to relax and calm their emotions.

1. Pretend to hand out a restaurant menu to the children.

2. Ask the children to choose their favourite hot food.

3. Bring the hands towards the nose.

4. Gently cup the hands open and pretend there is a bowl of your favourite food inside the hands.

5. Sniff and take short inhales through the nose to smell the delicious food.

6. Continue smelling the food for ten more seconds.

7. Inform the children the food is too hot to eat.

8. Blow through the mouth to cool the food down.

9. Repeat for two more rounds or for as long as necessary.

10. Imagine the food is now ready to eat: 'Hmmm, delicious!'

This activity can be adapted to smelling dandelion flowers through the nostrils with quick inhales (sniffing) and then blowing on to the flowers with the mouth using extended exhales.

Therapeutic Benefits

- Relaxes children and calms emotions
- Enhances creative imagination and thinking skills
- Strengthens hand–eye coordination
- Stimulates the senses

Developmental Skills

- Body awareness
- Fine motor
- Oral motor
- Cognitive learning
- Self-care and organisation

Be Mindful

Children can participate in this activity without the hands by simply focusing on the breath and imagining the objects. For greater impact and to reinforce the concept of breathing mindfully, use physical props or real food and/or flowers. Pictorial visual symbols can also be used as prompts to represent items.

Hot Air Balloon

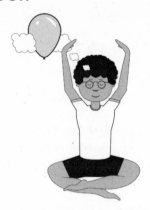

You will need...

- Optional: visuals to show balloons gliding through the air

- Optional: balloons to practice inhaling and exhaling

The floating sensation of balloons drifting through the air can create a calming experience for children. When children use the breath and their imagination to recreate floating balloons, it can help settle the mind and release pent-up feelings.

1. Sit in a comfortable position with the legs crossed and back straight.

2. Ask the children what colour their (imaginary) balloon is or show visuals of balloons and get them to choose their favourite colour.

3. Cup both hands around the mouth.

4. Exhale and blow out through the mouth.

5. Breathe in through the nose as the hands and arms are raised above the head in the shape of the balloon.

6. Pause for a few moments.

7. Inform the children that the balloon is being filled up with air and is helping them let go of unwanted thoughts and feelings.

8. Breathe out through the mouth as the arms lower towards the face.

9. Cup the hand around the mouth again.

10. Continue to breathe in and out in sync with the arms – moving up with every inhale through the nose and then down to the mouth with every exhale through the mouth.

11. With every inhale, the hands and arms should move wider apart when they are above the head to show the balloon is growing.

12. Remember to pause for a few moments every time the arms are raised.

13. Repeat for four more rounds. At the end of the last round, the arms should remain above the head – wide apart in the shape of a big hot air balloon.

14. Inform the children that the balloon is about to soar through the skies.

15. Sway the body (still seated) with the arms wide to one side as you breathe in and sway to the other side as you breathe out.

16. Continue until the children feel calm.

Ask children who do not like balloons to visualise and imagine other inflatable objects floating through the air, e.g. bubbles, spaceships and aeroplanes. Simplify the language and actions by modelling this activity and using visual picture symbols (if required) to support the children's understanding. As an alternative to cupping the hands around the mouth, children can also place their hands on the chest or the head as they exhale to create the mindful experience of releasing feelings from the heart space (hands on the chest) or thoughts from the mind (hands on the head). Once children are well versed in Balloon Breathing, at the end of the session, gently lower the arms and hands to the floor and imagine the balloon popping by patting the floor whilst making popping sounds.

Therapeutic Benefits

- Calms and relaxes the mind and body

- Enhances focus and concentration

- Builds upper body strength

- Improves hand–eye coordination

- Improves creative thinking skills

- Stimulates the senses

Developmental Skills

- Body awareness

- Gross motor

- Fine motor

- Cognitive learning

- Crosses the midline

- Self-care and organisation

- Planning and sequencing

Be Mindful

Children who are unable to remain in a crossed legged position can complete this activity sat in a chair or standing. Hand-over-hand support and encouragement may be required if children experience difficulties with fine motor, gross motor or sequencing skills. To enhance the senses, start the session by blowing up real balloons to touch and observe how they inflate and move, particularly with children who are unable to visualise or feeling anxious. Alternatively, watch a video clip of hot air balloons gliding through the air.

Mind Bubbles

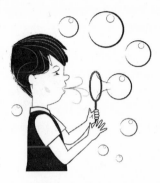

You will need...

- Bottle of bubbles

The simple act of blowing bubbles combined with mindfully visualising the letting go of unwanted thoughts and feelings can enhance a state of calm and release stress.

1. Take deep breaths in through the nose and extended exhales through the mouth.

2. Mindfully blow bubbles into the air.

3. Observe how the bubbles float up, down and around until each bubble pops.

4. Continue to take deep breaths.

5. Imagine the bubbles are negative thoughts from the mind or heavy emotions in the body.

6. Notice that blowing mind bubbles means that any busy thoughts or low feelings are no longer in the mind or body, because they are floating outside in the open air.

7. Every time the bubbles pop, it symbolises the letting go and moving on of the negative thoughts and feelings, which vanish into thin air.

8. Breathe in deeply to gently replace these feelings with peace, happiness, self-compassion and kindness from within.

9. Continue mindfully blowing bubbles, remembering to pause and observe the bubbles each time, until the children feel calm.

As an alternative to bubbles, children can place fine materials like sequins and rice in the hands or hold dandelion flowers to represent their negative thoughts and feelings. Blow on the materials and watch them float up into the air and then down onto the ground to represent the letting go and release of the thoughts and feelings.

Therapeutic Benefits

- Calms and relaxes the mind and body
- Improves focus and concentration
- Enhances creative thinking skills
- Improves self-esteem
- Improves hand–eye coordination
- Stimulates the senses (particularly auditory and tactile)

Developmental Skills

- Fine motor
- Oral motor
- Cognitive learning
- Self-care and organisation
- Visual perception and tracking
- Planning and sequencing

Be Mindful

Provide hand-over-hand support or use a bubble machine for children with fine motor and oral motor difficulties. Simplify the language as necessary to secure children's understanding.

The bubbles or materials that are blown can also symbolise positive emotions, like joy, happiness and love, that children would like to feel thankful for. Ask more cognitively able children to observe how the bubbles fall and float, the different shapes and sizes of bubbles and any sounds or sensations on the skin if they can feel or hear the bubbles pop on their body.

Guided Imagery with the Breath

You will need...

- Guided Imagery Scripts from Section 3 of Part V: Resources

- Optional: soft background music

In Guided Imagery, children use the power of their imagination to visualise positive mental images and find a sense of peace from within.

The two Guided Imagery scripts, Starfish and Sun Bliss, in Section 3 of Part V: Resources use the power of conscious breathing to instil a sense of calm in children.

If the children require help to visualise, present visual images or props, e.g. starfish, ocean, sunshine, pond, etc., before the children lie down and close their eyes.

Therapeutic Benefits

- Calms and relaxes the mind and body

- Enhances focus and concentration

- Develops social–emotional skills

- Improves the physiological and psychological state

- Stimulates the senses

Developmental Skills

- Body awareness

- Cognitive learning

- Self-care and organisation

- Planning and sequencing

Be Mindful

If it is not a distraction, play soft music in the background to help deepen the mind–body sensations. Adapt the language, characters and content of Guided Imagery to suit the children's level of understanding. Recording the session with a child's voice can also enhance this experience. Children can keep their eyes open if they do not feel comfortable closing them. In many cases, Guided Imagery can initially be practised as a physical drama activity by recreating the text of the imagery through physical movements. The children then close their eyes and focus on their breath to participate mindfully.

BODY FLOW

Synchronise the breath and stimulate the senses with mindful body movements.

Palming

Palming was originally created by an ophthalmologist in the early 1900s to improve eyesight. Today, Palming, which may initially resemble a game of 'peek a boo', offers a fun and warming way for children to gently rest the hands over the eyes and experience relaxation.

1. Sit or stand in a comfortable position with the back straight.

2. Rub the fingers and palms of both hands together in circular and vertical motions.

3. Mindfully count to 20 whilst rubbing the hands together.

4. Tilt the head and shoulders forward.

5. Close the eyes and cup the left hand over the left eye and right hand over the right eye.

6. Gently rest the head on the hands.

7. Keep the eyes closed.

8. Relax the shoulders and elbows down.

9. Deeply breathe in and out. Feel the warming sensations from the hands on the face as this enhances relaxation.

10. Continue to breathe deeply for 30 seconds with the hands cupped over the eyes.

11. If required, repeat for another round.

Once the children feel confident with Palming and experience the relaxing benefits, challenge them to make it as dark as possible and to keep the light out with their hands.

Therapeutic Benefits

- Calms the mind and enhances mental clarity

- Improves focus and brings the attention inwards

- Relaxes the facial muscles and upper body

- Improves hand–eye coordination

- Stimulates the senses (particularly tactile and visual)

Developmental Skills

- Body awareness

- Visual perception

- Fine motor

- Self-care and organisation

Be Mindful

Check that when the children cover their eyes with their hands, they use the least amount of pressure. Ensure the shoulders and arms are as loose as possible and support children with fine motor difficulties to hold their hands into position. Alternatively, yoga eye pads can be used alongside the deep breathing. For more able children, include Counting the Breath on page 28.

Log Roll

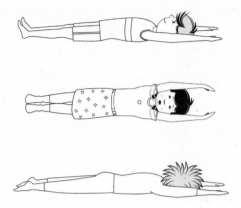

Log Roll is a playful and energising breathing activity, where children breathe mindfully whilst physically rolling the entire body.

1. Lay down comfortably with the back straight, legs together and arms by the side.

2. Take a deep breath in through the nose.

3. Breathe out with a long exhale through the mouth and roll the body for as long as the exhale.

4. When the body roll and simultaneous exhale end, pause to breathe in and out naturally for a few moments.

5. Take another deep breath in and continue with the actions above as many times as suitable.

When children become comfortable with the Log Roll, if suitable experiment by changing the rhythm of the breath with a long exhale as children lay still on their backs and a deep inhale as their bodies roll. Ask them if they notice any difference in how they feel.

Therapeutic Benefits

*   Creates a relaxing and reenergising effect

*   Gently massages the body and releases tension

- Strengthens the core and grounds the mind and body

- Enhances creative and social play skills

- Builds confidence and independence

- Stimulates the senses, particularly the vestibular sensory system

Developmental Skills

- Body awareness

- Gross motor

- Planning and sequencing

- Self-care and organisation

Be Mindful

For children who are unable to independently perform the body roll, ask them to focus on the inhale and long exhale of the breath as the adults physically move their body on their behalf. For children with weak muscle strength who want to independently perform this activity, encourage them to place their hands on the floor to push the body into the rolling motion. If rolling the body creates feelings of dizziness or overstimulation, pause or stop the activity. Be sure to set clear boundaries and use a visual timer if the children become over excited or hyperactive during this playful activity.

Personal Hug

The soothing sensation received from gentle hugs can be very calming for children. When the Personal Hug is linked to the breath, additional comfort and feelings of warmth and safety are created.

1. Sit or stand in a comfortable position.

2. Breathe in through the nose as the arms and hands open out in front of the body at shoulder height.

3. Create a balloon shape with the arms.

4. Breathe out and place the hands on opposite shoulders.

5. Hug the shoulders.

6. Squeeze and push the hands on the shoulders.

7. Continue for as many rounds as is required.

Therapeutic Benefits

- Gently massages and releases tension from the body

- Builds self-esteem and independence

- Enhances relaxation and brings the attention inwards

- Improves hand–eye coordination

- Stimulates the senses

Developmental Skills

- Body awareness

- Fine motor

- Visual perception

- Crosses the midline

- Self-care and organisation

Be Mindful

For any children experiencing hypersensitivity, personal hugs may trigger defensive reactions, so find alternative breathing activities in this chapter tailored to their needs. If children find hugging themselves a challenge, particularly if they are unable to cross the midline, the Sensory Cuddle Swing on page 45 can be used instead, as this generates similar sensations to a human hug and is linked to the breath.

Tap Breathing

Tap Breathing is a 'muscle tense and release' body awareness exercise. The children tense muscle groups and then release the tension with the exhale of the breath. This creates the relaxed feeling of letting go of stress from within the body and refocuses the mind.

1. Stand with the legs together and back straight.

2. Raise the arms to shoulder height at either side of the body.

3. Create a T shape with the body.

4. Scrunch up the face.

5. Tighten the shoulders and arms and make fists with the hands.

6. Breathe in deeply through the nose.

7. Immediately breathe out through the mouth with a long exhale, creating a 'shhhhh' noise with a sigh that sounds like a tap releasing air.

8. Release the tension from the face, shoulders, arms and fists during the exhale.

9. Inform the children that the tap has let go of all the trapped air and pent-up energy.

10. Repeat for four more rounds.

11. Pause with the arms down to notice the sensations in the body and return to a natural breath.

Therapeutic Benefits

- Relieves tension from the upper body

- Focuses the mind and invigorates the body

- Stretches and builds strength in the body

- Builds self-esteem and confidence

- Stimulates the senses

Developmental Skills

- Body awareness

- Gross motor

- Fine motor

- Oral motor and phonological awareness

- Auditory discrimination

- Planning and sequencing

Be Mindful

Ensure that releasing the breath with the muscles has a continual flow by encouraging children not to hold on to the breath, as this may create added tension. Provide support as necessary for children who are unable to independently balance in the T position. This breathing activity can also be practised from a seated position. With non-verbal children, adults can create the sound effect or use pre-recorded sound to simulate the sound of the tap releasing air. For a full-body Progressive Relaxation activity, see the script in Section 4 of Part V: Resources.

Wall Push Ups

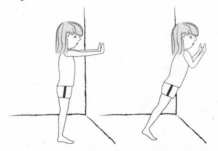

You will need...

- Sturdy wall or hard flat, vertical surface

Wall Push Ups connect physical exercise with the flow of the breath. Synchronising the breath with mindful movements calms the mind and builds upper body strength.

1. Stand in front of a blank wall with the back straight.

2. Ensure the feet are two to three footprints away from the wall and shoulder width apart.

3. Raise the arms to shoulder level and place the palms against the wall with the hands slightly wider apart than the shoulders.

4. Breathe in through the nose as the elbows gradually bend and the body moves towards the wall.

5. Blow out through mouth with a long exhale as the arms straighten and the body returns to the starting position.

6. Ensure the elbows are slightly bent on the outstretched arms.

7. Breathe in and out in sync with the bending and outstretching of the arms.

8. Keep the hands firmly in place on the wall at all times during this activity.

9. Continue for five to ten rounds, depending on the children's physical ability.

Once the children have become familiar with this activity, include a count of the push ups every time they exhale. For added fun, and if the children feel comfortable and have the upper body strength, bring their attention to the breath by changing the pace and rhythm of the push ups.

Therapeutic Benefits

- Focuses and calms the mind

- Strengthens the core and other muscles in the body

- Opens the chest and relieves tension

- Centres and grounds the body and mind

- Stimulates the senses

Developmental Skills

- Body awareness

- Fine motor

- Gross motor

- Self-care and organisation

- Planning and sequencing

Be Mindful

Encourage the children to keep the chest open, elbows soft and back as straight as possible when they participate in Wall Push Ups. Provide verbal prompts and reminders to focus on the breath with every physical arm movement. For children who have low muscle tone and/or are unable to independently balance and lean against the wall, consult an occupational therapist or physiotherapist for guidance before commencing this activity.

Rainbow Breathing

You will need...

- Visuals of rainbows

Rainbow breathing is a fun and calming activity to help children connect to the breath whilst stretching the arms above the head and creating imaginary rainbows.

1. Sit or stand in a comfortable position with the back straight and the feet firmly on the ground.

2. Relax the arms down by the side with the palms facing outwards.

3. It's now time to create some nice big rainbows. Ask the children what colours are in rainbows or show visuals of rainbows.

4. Keep the arms straight and slowly raise both arms upwards from the side.

5. Allow the arms to meet above the head when they get to the top in an extended prayer position.

6. Keep the hands in extended prayer position above the head and turn the wrists outwards towards the sides of the room.

7. Slowly lower the arms back down to the side of the body. That's the first rainbow!

8. Close the eyes this time, and prepare to imagine the colours of the next rainbow.

9. Breathe in through the nose as the arms slowly raise with the hands facing outwards. Remember to think of the colours of the rainbow and allow the arms to gently meet in the middle above the head.

10. Breathe out through the nose as the arms move back down and return to the starting position.

11. Make three more rainbows, and each time see if the arms can stretch out even wider.

In addition to the activity above, children may enjoy standing up and slowly moving into different areas in defined spaces to create the rainbows. To simplify this activity, particularly to help calm children after or during heightened emotional situations, raise the hands with the inhale and keep the hands above the head in prayer position during the exhale to continue deep breathing with the arms raised, and then gently lower the hands before creating another rainbow.

Therapeutic Benefits

- Focuses and calms the mind

- Improves hand–eye coordination
- Opens the chest and strengthens the muscles in the core and upper body
- Enhances an energised state
- Stimulates the senses

Developmental Skills

- Body awareness
- Fine motor
- Gross motor
- Self-care and organisation
- Planning and sequencing

Be Mindful

Encourage children to keep the chest open, elbows soft and back straight throughout the activity. Remind children to go slowly with this activity, as they may want to rush into creating rainbows. Support any children with hand–eye coordination or fine/gross motor difficulties by providing hand-over-hand support and prompts, or adults can model the activity whilst children observe and breathe in and out in sync with the movement of the adults' arms. Simplify the language and actions by modelling this activity and using visual picture symbols (if required) to support children's understanding.

Next Steps

When children learn to mindfully breathe, and how to let go, the body and mind naturally begin to relax. In the next chapter, we will explore the third part of the S.T.A.R. model and empower children by giving them additional tools with which to self-regulate.

Part II

And...

S	**Stop** what you are doing, gently drop your shoulders and allow yourself to be present in this moment.
T	**Take** some deep breaths as you close your eyes. Focus on your breathing (Chapter 3) and how this gradually helps you feel calm.
A	**And...** Pause for a few moments to observe your thoughts and feelings as you begin to feel more at peace.
R	**Relax**, let go and allow any thoughts and feelings to pass through your mind and body. Take time to gradually gain a more calming state of flow (Chapter 4).

Chapter 4

Self-Regulate and Flow

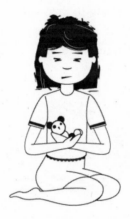

Children with special needs often require support to acquire and develop skills to process, adapt and monitor their thoughts, behaviours and emotions. This is particularly during transitions or when faced with new and unexpected situations. Therefore, the development of self-regulation by using practical tools and activities with children is imperative for their social, emotional and mental well-being.

Why Teach Children Self-Regulation?

Self-regulation tools in essence empower children to take back control using a grounded, self-reflective approach with the view of becoming more self-assured and independent. If used regularly, self-regulation tools enable children to feel calm and be more present, which can instil a sense of 'flow' into their everyday lives.

The mindful breathing activities in Chapter 3 are a form of self-regulation. Teaching children with special needs how to self-regulate, particularly during times of heightened emotions, can enhance a state of calm and then ease the transition between different experiences, improve communication skills and enable children to think for themselves and learn to resolve conflicts.

Many children with special needs feel overwhelmed by expectations placed upon them to conform and sit still for periods of time, listen attentively, follow routines, process information quickly and build relationships. Self-regulation and executive functioning skills are the process of children monitoring how they feel at any given time and then adapting to plan and make informed decisions that affect their thoughts, behaviour and emotions in accordance with experiences and immediate situations they find themselves in. This all begins within the brain.

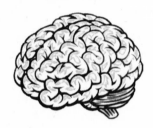

Upstairs Downstairs Brain

To help parents and educators understand the inner workings of children's brains, Dr Daniel Siegel and Dr Tina Payne Bryson describe the 'upstairs' and 'downstairs' parts of the brain in their book *The Whole-Brain Child* (2012). In children, particularly those with special needs, the brain is still developing or could be, in fact, underdeveloped. This can result in impulsive behaviour, poor working memory, lack of empathy and an inability to control their emotions and body.

Forebrain **Cerebral cortex** *Upstairs brain* Executive centre	**Limbic brain, hindbrain amygdala,** **cerebellum, brainstem** *Downstairs brain* Emotional centre and alarm centre
Higher order thinking: • Planning • Decision making • Impulse control • Imagining • Analytical thinking • Logic • Body and emotional regulation • Self-understanding	Acts out of instinct: • Flight, fight or freeze • Motivation • Memory • Attachment • Motor regulation • Balance • Blinking • Breathing/heart rate • Heart rate • Blood pressure
Integrate the upstairs and downstairs brain with a metaphorical staircase Develop executive function and self-regulation skills	

As shown in the table above, children need input from both parts of the brain in order to make informed decisions and regulate their emotions. For example, if a child is scared of the dark, this may trigger feelings of fear and anxiety ('downstairs' brain). However, if a metaphoric 'higher thinking' staircase is in place going towards the 'upstairs brain', the child learns how to self-regulate and make the informed decision to turn the light on in the room and seek reassurance from an adult. See Flipping Your Lid on page 143 for guidance on how to simplify and explain the upstairs downstairs brain to children.

When the brain is functioning, it can help children plan, focus, coordinate tasks, process sensory input and store information in the subconscious mind. Executive function ('upstairs' brain) and self-regulation ('downstairs' brain) are the brain's mechanisms to activate self-control, mental flexibility and working memory. Therefore, in order for children to make wise decisions, remember instructions and regulate emotions, the 'upstairs' and 'downstairs' parts of the brain need to work in cohesion.

Being in the Zone

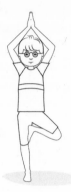

When children achieve a state of flow, they are in a mental state of 'being in the zone'. There is no resistance or thoughts of the past or future, because the present moment is all that matters, along with being fully absorbed and in the flow of the activity. By pursuing their passions and being in a flow state on a regular basis, children improve their mental capacity to: concentrate for longer periods of time; feel at peace and self-assured; have a sense of achievement; be less stressed; and be creative.

Connecting Self-Regulation to Being in the Flow

Self-regulation and being in the flow go hand in hand. By learning to self-regulate, children develop empowering skills to live in the present moment and take ownership of their emotional state, thoughts and behaviours without placing judgement upon them. Once children are in the present moment, they are in the perfect mind-set to simply be themselves and develop a sense of flow by connecting to their breath, feeling the sensations in their body and placing their full attention on what they are doing. Activities with a natural sense of flow can include laughing with loved ones, fun 'brain breaks', singing, painting, walking or anything that inspires and fully engages the child.

Often, when children receive additional adult support to self-regulate in the classroom, they may not want the attention to be drawn towards them, as it could highlight how different they are from their classmates, so be mindful of initiating the following tools with an element of discretion. This can result in meltdowns and bouts of anxiety and frustration.

Whilst there are several self-regulation activities that can enhance a state of flow, this chapter focuses on the following types of activity due to their benefits for regulating children special needs.

- Grounding

- Sensory yoga

- Emotional intelligence

- Lego®-based therapy

- Calm Down Jar

- Music therapy

Each technique mindfully instils self-awareness and essential tools to self-calm and helps develop the social, emotional and mental well-being of all children.

GROUNDING

Grounding, also known as earthing, is a self-regulation technique that encourages children to become aware of the surface beneath their feet and connect to the earth's grounding energy. This helps calm the nervous system, brings their bodily sensations and attention into the present and creates a balanced state of mind. The 54321 Grounding technique is a sensory awareness tool that can be done in a variety of settings, in isolation or alongside other self-regulation techniques.

Steps to 54321 Grounding

Visual
5 things you can see.

Tactile
4 things you can feel or touch.

Auditory
3 things you can hear.

Olfactory
2 things you can smell.

Interoception
1 thing you like about yourself or an emotion you can feel. This includes internal body sensations.

Read out each step to the children, pausing after each one to let them notice the things you are asking them to look for. During each step, use a calming tone of voice with minimal language. Encourage the children to have their eyes open so they are alert, remain in one space with their feet on the ground (if possible) and respond clearly to your instructions, as this helps to keep them present. Hold the space in a neutral, non-judgemental manner and calmly guide children to respond naturally with the first things they notice. As the children progress through the sensory systems, simplify the language or use visual picture cues to support the level of understanding.

When children use the senses to notice their surroundings in a non-judgemental way using the visual, tactile, auditory and olfactory sensory systems, and then gradually hone in on themselves in that present moment with interoception, they can develop a sense of inner connection and closure to the grounding process that facilitates a mindful transition to the next activity in a state of flow. Ending on one thing the children like about themselves can help enhance self-image and connection from within.

The original 54321 format ends with one thing children can taste (gustatory); this has been adapted to a mindfulness approach for children with special needs.

Grounding with Progressive Relaxation

You will need...

- Grounding with Progressive Relaxation script from Section 4 of Part V: Resources

- Optional: soft background music

Progressive Relaxation is a body awareness and relaxation tool that grounds and calms children, particularly when experiencing heightened emotions. Progressive Relaxation involves tensing and relaxing the muscles with the breath, which helps reduce physiological problems and improves sleep.

Read the Progressive Relaxation script in Section 4 of Part V: Resources slowly and calmly. Ensure the children lie down or sit in a comfortable position with straight backs. If the children are seated, ensure both feet are placed flat on the ground.

Progressive Relaxation can be adapted towards children's physical needs and level of understanding. Adding music or recording the session with the children's voices can be a way to enhance the experience.

When they are participating in Progressive Relaxation as a grounding activity, ensure the children do not tense the muscles with their full strength, as this may cause pain and/or heighten feelings of anxiety. They should also *avoid holding the breath* and should simply squeeze the muscles with the in breath and then release the tension with the exhale, as this encourages a natural flow of breath whilst enhancing body awareness.

SENSORY YOGA

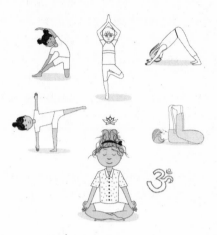

The word 'yoga' comes from the Sanskrit root yuj, which means 'to yoke' or join together the mind, body and spirit. Yoga is an ancient practice of meditation, conscious breathing, stretching, moving into postures and, ultimately, finding peace from within. The practice can: bring a sense of calm; increase strength and flexibility; develop self-awareness; balance the mind-set; and be grounding for children with special needs. Yogis are encouraged to listen to their hearts and find their true paths in life. As a combination of mindfulness and awareness of the whole body, yoga encourages yogis to see the practice as a way of living a self-aware, peaceful and compassionate life beyond the yoga mat.

Children with special needs may, on occasion, require support to regulate the amount of sensory information presented to them at any given time. The human body has eight main sensory systems that affect how external stimulus is processed and regulated by the brain, which then results in corresponding motor and behavioural responses. The sensory systems are gustatory (taste), tactile (touch), olfactory (smell), visual (sight), auditory (sound), vestibular (movement and balance), proprioceptive (body awareness) and interoceptive (internal bodily sensations).

The term 'sensory overload' often refers to children feeling overstimulated by receiving too much sensory input, e.g. flashing lights, loud noises or bright colours. Children with 'sensory under-responsiveness' may require additional sensory input due to the brain being slow to respond to sensory information presented to them, e.g. they may not feel pain or be able to differentiate between strong tastes and or they may have weak muscles. In addition, 'sensory craving' may occur when children constantly seek sensory input because they feel something is lacking from particular sensory systems, e.g. always hugging others, repeatedly making noises or watching the same music video clip over and over again. It should also be noted that there are other forms of sensory processing disorder, but sensory yoga is a proven therapeutic method that can help children with special needs to self-regulate and find a sense of balance and flow in each moment (Collins, 2015).

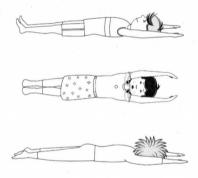

Teaching children with special needs simple yoga movements using a step-by-step visual schedule can give them an incredibly empowering form of self-regulation and sensory integration. Sensory integration is the neurological process in which the brain absorbs sensory information from the body and environment, processes this and then organises the information to provide a response.

Children are asked to breathe mindfully whilst doing the movements so they notice their bodies' sensations – what they can see, hear, smell and feel. Reassure them in a calm and non-judgemental way that it's okay to experience and recognise these sensations. Sensory props and activities including fairy lights, blowing bubbles, weighted blankets, playdough, soft balls to squeeze, creating human massage trains, listening to musical instruments and creating mindful movements linked to breathing can be used to help ground and centre children with special needs.

Yoga Games

Simple yoga games, visuals and storytelling help children with special needs live in the moment, engage the sensory system and enhance creative play skills.

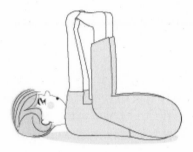

ॐ Yoga and Storytelling

You will need...

- Yoga Story Script from Section 5 of Part V: Resources

- Yoga cards (e.g. *The Yogi! Card Set*, Hughes, 2017)

Storytelling is a popular way to lead children through and teach a yoga sequence. Yoga stories often carry messages to remind children of their qualities and to practice gratitude, show compassion, be kind to themselves and others and even understand more abstract concepts like seasons of the year, emotions and events.

Section 5 of Part V: Resources contains Josie the Star, an interactive yoga story script to read to children. This story can be adapted to suit different levels of understanding, particularly if visual picture cues for additional support are required.

ॐ Sensory Wrap and Roll

You will need...

- Yoga mat, soft blanket, towel or spandex

Many children with special needs are supported to regulate their senses. The Sensory Wrap and Roll is a body awareness activity that can help calm the nervous system during times of heighted emotions or wake a child up when they are feeling tired or low.

Ask the child to lay their body at one end of a yoga mat, soft blanket, towel or spandex, as these materials help provide even tactile pressure. Tell the child they are going to be rolled up like a tasty pancake with their body as the lovely filling, which can be any food they like. Rhythmically wrap and roll the child's body into the whole piece of material from their shoulders down to the feet. Wrapping the child with the material helps him or her to physically feel together, safe and grounded, and it calms the mind and body. Next, ask the child again about the flavour of the pancake and pretend to eat it. Lastly, when the child feels calm, inform him or her that they are about to be unwrapped. Gently, safely and swiftly unwrap the material. The swift tactile action rolls the whole body out of the fabric and helps the child become alert and ready to move on.

Yoga Visuals

Yoga cards (for example, *The Go Yogi! Card Set*, Hughes, 2017) offer children with special needs visual support and facilitate an inclusive approach towards learning. Visuals help children focus, make abstract learning more concrete and can enhance social communication. Yoga cards show images of people in yoga poses and do a great job of reinforcing the holistic learning experience of yoga. Here, we will focus on yoga games – a self-regulation tool – using yoga cards.

৺ Yoga Dice

You will need...

- Large sensory dice or dice with pockets to insert your own yoga visuals

Dice rolling is an ancient recreational pastime often used today in board games, academic learning and other activities to stimulate and engage the mind. The unpredictable outcome of rolling a die gives players a sense of anticipation, drive and suspense. In this game, choose six different yoga pose cards and number each with a whiteboard pen from one to six. Put the yoga cards in places that are easy to reach and see around the room or space. Next, the children should take turns to roll the die and wait to see what number it lands on. Ask them to go the yoga card with the corresponding number and use their bodies to match the card's yoga poses. For small groups, and depending on the level of understanding, you can use two dice for different children to roll simultaneously. Continue to take turns and offer support as necessary.

৺ Yoga Card Game

You will need...

- Yoga cards (e.g. *The Go Yogi! Card Set*, Hughes, 2017)

To initiate this game, the adult should show three yoga cards to the children. Next, the adult should move their own body into one of the yoga positions from a card and then ask the children to choose the card to match the pose. Everyone then performs the yoga pose together. The adult continues until all three of the positions and cards have been demonstrated. After the card game has been modelled by the adult, children can take turns at leading with the cards, with everyone else choosing the matching cards with the poses to move into together. Once children are confident in playing this game, adapt and modify as necessary.

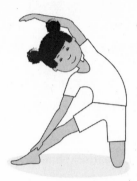

ॐ Musical Yogi

You will need...

- Pre-recorded sounds (e.g. piano, ocean, birds, lullabies, flutes)

- Musical instruments for live music

- Audio device

- Yoga cards (e.g. *The Go Yogi! Card Set*, Hughes, 2017)

Play calming or uplifting music to reflect how you would like the children to feel. Dance along to the music with the children. If a child is not comfortable with dancing, ask him or her to gently sway or slowly walk around a defined space. Stop the music after a minute and demonstrate a yoga pose for the children to copy and mirror back to you. Help the children move into the postures as necessary. Depending on the level of understanding, after the pose, show two yoga cards – one card with the yoga pose they just practised and the other card with a different yoga pose. Ask the children to choose and take the card with the yoga pose they just moved into; then, if it's appropriate, as they look at the yoga card ask them how this made them feel. Calmly reassure the children that any feelings they may have are okay. It's important to simply have fun. Restart the music and continue this practice with different poses.

EMOTIONAL INTELLIGENCE

Mindfulness can be achieved by encouraging children to be aware of their emotions and teaching them to allow their emotions to arise without judging them. Emotions are conscious, moving experiences creating physiological, mental and feeling sensations. The word 'emotion' means energy in motion. Emotions therefore affect children's behaviour and how they experience the world around them. When children and young people learn how to manage their feelings, they develop greater self-esteem, become better problem solvers and are more equipped to deal with unexpected situations.

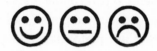

Many children with special needs receive support to regulate their emotional states, particularly during transitions and busy times because these can trigger heightened emotions including anxiety and frustration. Teaching emotional intelligence to children is vital because it gives them the ability to recognise and manage their own emotions and also the emotions of others. This happens when children learn how to develop emotional awareness by gaining the knowledge to adapt their emotional state in relation to specific tasks and situations and learning how to use empathy to regulate their own emotions and help others to calm down or cheer up.

It is vital for children with special needs to develop an understanding that every emotional state they experience is part of being human. Everyone has great days, good days and not-so-great days; and, as children go through the ups, downs and roundabouts of each day, their emotions ebb and flow. Whenever a child is feeling sad, anxious, happy, angry, frustrated, nervous, apprehensive and so forth, emotional regulation can help him or her neutrally recognise these emotions, regulate their state and process this in a non-judgemental way.

Emotional Awareness

Emotions can range from frustrated to elated, angry to calm, tired to energised and so forth. Emotional awareness in children is the practice of identifying and expressing how they feel and is a useful self-regulation tool that can develop a sense of compassion and self-awareness. Whilst developing emotional awareness, many children say they feel either happy or sad when talking about their emotions, when actually they may be excited or frustrated but do not have the emotional skills to express this.

Emotions journals help children understand the natural ebb and flow of emotions and how to access their emotions without judging them. Using a physical book to write, draw or stick visuals in is preferable, if it's appropriate to the children's needs, because it provides a tangible sensory tool that enhances creativity and triggers the memory recall and retention parts of the brain. This in turn develops critical thinking, conceptual development and comprehension. For children who experience fine motor difficulties, provide hand-over-hand support and a choice of visuals to stick into the book.

Journaling

Journaling in a physical book can be a useful way to develop emotional awareness in children. The activity below sets out how to help children to create an emotions journal.

1. Introduce and talk about a specific emotion (e.g. nervousness) using emotion cards for visual prompts (e.g. *The Mood Cards* by Andrea Harrn, 2015).

2. Ask the children to explore what this emotion means to them.

3. Ask the children to draw pictures, write notes or stick visuals in the journals to represent what this emotion looks like from their perspectives (see Section 6 of Part V: Resources). Be creative, and remember – there is no right or wrong.

4. Discuss the images placed or drawn in the journal.

5. Ask the children to think of real-life situations where they have experienced this emotion.

6. Focus on three calming strategies children can do to self-regulate when they feel this emotion, e.g. animal breathing, sensory yoga, building with Lego®.

7. Draw, stick visuals or write a list of these calming strategies in the journal.

8. Discuss the calming strategies and develop a daily routine of reviewing the content in the journal.

Encourage the children to journal and express how they feel every day. Activities such as drawing faces to represent different emotions and creating calming strategy visuals as shown in Section 6 of Part V: Resources can be used with the emotions journal to help children self-reflect, develop emotional literacy and connect more deeply with their emotions.

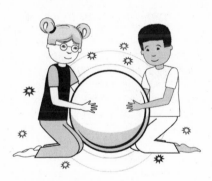

Emotional Regulation

Emotional regulation has been described as the 'the intra and extra organismic factors by which emotional arousal is redirected, controlled, modulated and modified to enable an individual to function adaptively' (Cicchetti, Ganiban and Barnett, 1991: 15). Equipping children with techniques to help regulate their emotions can develop their capacity to: **independently self-regulate** using sensory, cognitive and/or linguistic strategies; **mutually regulate** by seeking regulatory support from trusted adults/peers and responding appropriately; and **recover from dysregulation** – extreme emotional states in which children are supported to function using mutual regulation so they eventually learn to self-regulate. The following steps provide guidance to support a child with special needs through dysregulation:

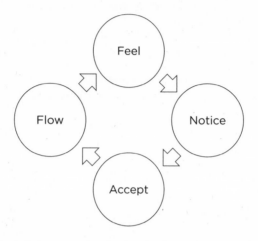

> **You will need...**
>
> • Emotion cards and other emotion visuals (e.g. traffic light think fan)
>
> • Book to write, draw or stick visuals of emotions in
>
> • Faces of Emotion sheet from Section 7 of Part V: Resources

Step One: Self Compassion – Feel

It's important to give children the time and space to experience their emotions, provided they are safe and it causes no harm to themselves or others. When they are ready, calmly talk with them or show visuals to help them describe how they are feeling. Reassure and inform the children that it's okay to feel how they feel and give them time to connect to their emotions. Encourage children to use self-compassion as they notice the emotions that come up for them. Be patient and provide a safe space for children to feel and express their emotions in a calm and neutral manner. Move on to the next step only when you feel children are ready to focus for a few moments and be engaged in visual stimuli.

Step Two: Non-Judgement – Notice

Colour-coded and pictorial symbols, like emotion cards, are useful tools to help children identify and label their emotions. Labelling emotions: engages the brain; enables children to gradually quell their emotional state; and empowers them to accept their present state and move forward.

Depending on the children's sensory, cognitive and linguistic reasoning, visuals or props can be created to represent different emotive colour codes. For example: **red** for angry emotions; **blue** for sad emotions; **yellow** for anxious/nervous emotions; and **green** for calm/happy. An alternative could be to use the weather to represent the emotions: **thunder** for angry emotions; **rain** for sad emotions; **cloud** for anxious/nervous emotions; and **sunshine** for calm/happy emotions. For a more simplistic approach, use **sad**, **neutral** and **happy** faces or sensory toys like 'feeling buddies', which show different facial expressions for emotions.

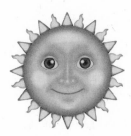

Ask the children to choose the visual to match and label how they feel. This may take time and will require patience on your part. Calmingly reassure children that it's okay to feel how they feel, because every emotion is okay and perfectly valid, and that admitting their emotional state makes them stronger.

Step Three: Inner Power – Accept

Once the children start to become calmer and more accepting of their emotional state, help them become responsible for their behaviour and take their power back by offering a choice between two or three self-regulating strategies and asking them to choose one. If the children are unable to choose a strategy for themselves, choose a strategy on their behalf. These strategies could be as simple as using the breathing exercises in Chapter 3, drinking a glass of water, listening to music on headphones, heavy work activities, jumping on the trampoline for five minutes, talking to an adult or going for a walk. Whatever they choose, the calming strategy should help children accept and move through their heightened emotions both internally and externally to eventually return to a peaceful state.

Step Four: Self-Reflect – Let Go and Flow!

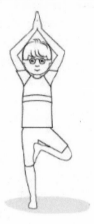

Lastly, to develop an inner sense of flow, return to the visuals in Step Two and ask the children to feel the sensations and label their current emotion. Reflect and commend the children for mindfully taking their power back by choosing a regulating tool that has helped them move through their emotions. It can take time for some children to genuinely recognise and label their emotional state, so reassure them that this is okay. If children continue to experience uncomfortable emotions, use a visual timetable to schedule in regular calming strategies throughout each day. Once achieved, emotional regulation can be incredibly self-fulfilling for children, resulting in emotions that gradually flow from within and create life-affirming experiences.

Emotional intelligence equips children with the tools not only to recognise and regulate emotions in themselves, but also to recognise how emotions can affect other people. With mindful practice children gradually develop empathy and the compassion to help regulate the emotional state of others.

LEGO®-BASED THERAPY

LEGO® was created in the late 1940s by a Danish toy company to encourage children to 'play well'. Today, LEGO® is a popular pastime for children and adults alike. The simple act of connecting interlocking bricks and shapes and then building new structures can be an incredibly fulfilling experience.

LEGO® enables children to work independently or with others during informal sessions to interlock and build objects; use their creativity and imagination or visual prompts for inspiration; observe colours, shapes, animals, and other features; and notice different emotional states with LEGO® faces. In essence, LEGO® can be used to positively distract, calm and self-regulate children in many different ways.

LEGO® can develop the skills that many children with special needs find difficult. These include collaborative play, fine motor skills, hand–eye coordination, visual perception, self-esteem, emotional literacy, communication, perseverance, problem solving, numeracy skills and creativity.

Due to the immense benefit and simplicity of LEGO®, Dr LeGoff, an American neuropsychologist, explored its use as a social, behaviour and cognitive intervention tool for children on the autistic spectrum and with neurodevelopmental disabilities. LEGO®-Based Therapy was created to help children enhance social communication through: collaborative play; self-control; turn-taking; sharing ideas; listening and attention skills; speech and language; and many other aspects of social communication.

When participating in LEGO®-Based Therapy, children gradually adapt their behaviour and emotional state to work in a group towards a shared focus. In the book *LEGO®-Based Therapy* by Simon Baron-Cohen *et al.*, it was noted that as children participate in the skill-building approach, their current 'social and adaptive functioning, self-regulation, and problem-solving, stereotypies and social deficits are replaced by more adaptive communicative gestures or self-regulatory gestures in all relevant settings' (2014: 32). Therefore, with clear rules and boundaries put in place at the start of sessions, e.g. 'use indoor voices' and 'if you can't fix it, ask for help', Lego®-Based Therapy can be viewed as a practical self-regulation tool.

LEGO®-Based Therapy sessions, better known as LEGO® Clubs to children, are conducted by trained facilitators, usually speech and language therapists, and supported by specialist teachers, other therapists or parents. Although parents and other professionals are encouraged to participate in sessions, and to continue similar activities with children away from the sessions, they should seek guidance from a trained facilitator beforehand to experience the full benefit of self-regulation.

LEGO® Club in Action

You will need...

- LEGO® pieces
- Images of objects made out of LEGO®
- Timer
- Emotion cards and other emotion visuals (e.g. traffic light think fan)

1. Ensure children of a similar age range are in a comfortable setting suitable for building and exploring LEGO®.

2. Group the children into threes, with one adult per group.

3. Assign the roles of 'architect' (also known as the 'engineer'), 'supplier' and 'builder' to each child.

4. Hand the architect a visual of a simple object made out of Lego® (for examples of visuals see Lego® Therapy by Drinkwater-Burke, 2016). The architect hides this visual from the rest of the group during the activity.

5. The supplier and architect collect the pieces from the main LEGO® box. Alternatively, for lower ability groups, give the architect the correct amount/colours/size of LEGO® pieces when they receive the visual.

6. As a team, the children work together to build and create the object on the visual out of LEGO®.

   - The architect instructs and guides the supplier on which LEGO® pieces to select, without pointing or directly showing them.

   - The supplier hands the LEGO® pieces to the builder after listening carefully to the instructions from the architect. The supplier may ask the architect questions for clarification.

   - The builder builds the object or model by using self-control to wait patiently for the Lego® pieces, listening and following the instructions from the architect on how to construct the model. The builder may also ask the architect questions for clarification.

7. Once the LEGO® model has been created, the children celebrate their achievement and reflect.

   - What did my team make out of LEGO®?

   - What did I enjoy most about this task?

   - What did I find tricky?

   - Have I given my team members a celebratory high five?

8. If appropriate, switch the roles to ensure each child experiences the activity from a different perspective and builds upon the social communication skillsets.

Due to the shared-attention and systematic-reasoning elements, LEGO® Club can be highly motivating for children, particularly if the visuals of objects have been carefully chosen to relate to the children's personal interests.

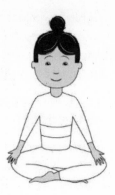

Adapt any of the steps above to facilitate inclusive access, particularly with children who have differing cognitive abilities, struggle with self-control and/or require additional assistance with social communication. For instance, replace the reflection questions with smiley face visuals for low ability children, use a visual egg timer or 'wait' visual symbol to reinforce the concept of turn-taking or provide more complex Lego® model visuals for gifted and talented children.

Regular use of LEGO® through child-initiated play or carefully guided collaboration with others over time will help children build self-regulation skills, improve their verbal and non-verbal communication, boost their social skills and enhance their self-esteem.

CALM DOWN JAR

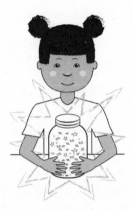

Calm Down Jars are used as a calming strategy for children during times of anxiety, stress or other heightened emotions. Calm Down Jars tend to contain water, glitter glue, food colouring and sequins. The jar's contents represent children's thoughts and feelings. For greater impact, encourage children to participate in the highly tactile and kinaesthetic process of making of the Calm Down Jar.

You will need...

- Empty clean jar
- Lid for Calm Down Jar
- Emotion cards and other emotion visuals (e.g. traffic light think fan)
- Water
- Glitter glue
- Food colouring
- Sequins
- Any other sparkly, floating materials

To make a Calm Down Jar

1. Add warm water to a jar until it is half full.

2. Squirt glitter glue into the water and stir the mixture.

3. Add a small amount of food colouring.

4. Sprinkle some glitter into the water (not too much – so there's enough room for the glitter to swirl).

5. Stir the mixture together.

6. Add the remaining water so the jar is now full.

7. Allow time for the water to cool down.

8. Screw the lid onto the jar with glue. *For children's safety, it would be advisable to use a plastic jar and ensure the lid is permanently screwed.*

Watching the shiny particles drift, float and gradually settle can be incredibly soothing for children, whilst directing their attention towards a focal point and stimulating the senses.

Calm Down Jar

1. To participate, find a comfortable space to sit or stand and then place the jar on a flat surface.

2. Mindfully breathe in and out for the count of five each time.

3. Shake the glitter jar hard and fast. Observe the shiny particles moving and swirling around the jar in many different directions. These particles can be feelings of frustration, confusion, anger, anxiety and so forth.

4. Continue to observe the particles in the jar and continue to breathe deeply to the count of five.

Children begin to notice the sparkles gradually settle within the jar. This experience can be calming and focusing, enhance feelings of contentment, relaxation and joy and soothe and balance the mind and being.

Ensure children are supervised at all times during this activity and that the jar lid is firmly fastened and secured with glue. Give the appropriate amount of verbal and visual instruction to support the level of understanding, as too much verbal input may be overwhelming. In many cases, just shaking and watching the Calm Down Jars settle with no verbal input will suffice. If children are unable to grip and shake the Calm Down Jars for themselves, adults can shake on their behalf or provide hand-over-hand support. Encourage more able children to verbalise or show visuals to represent how they feel at the end of the Calm Down Jar process.

MUSIC THERAPY

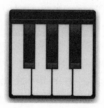

Music is a powerful channel for creativity, heritage and culture. Studies show that listening to music for an hour a day over the course of a week can decrease pain, anxiety and depression, whilst increasing feelings of self-esteem and independence and enhancing self-awareness (Harvard Medical School, 2018). Music therapy is a multisensory clinical intervention tool often used to help children with special needs process psychological, emotional, cognitive, physical, communicative and social difficulties.

In music therapy, when children listen to and feel the rhythm and harmonies of live and recorded compositions, the music therapist facilitates a safe and interactive space to connect children with their inner feelings, form bonds with others, develop self-expression and create positive changes in their emotional well-being and communication.

As a highly-regarded self-regulation tool, music therapy: intervenes to help stimulate brainwaves that lead to meditative calming states, alertness or concentrated thinking; releases dopamine, a 'feel-good' chemical into the brain; occupies the mind and body with familiar and soothing sensations; acts as a distractor to take children away from negative stimuli; and can help reduce perceptions of pain, anxiety, disability and depression within children.

When a child plays a musical instrument, it engages and strengthens both hemispheres of the brain, particularly the visual, auditory and motor cortices. In turn, playing a tangible musical instrument can ignite children's creativity, logical thought processes and self-discipline and enhance fine motor skills. For a child, being handing a drum to beat, shaker to shake or another musical instrument of their choice to play with freely without judgement or condition can be a liberating and expressive playful experience. When children play musical instruments, the sensory system is stimulated as shown in the following table.

 Tactile: Feel the surface and different textures on parts of the instrument.

 Auditory: Listen to the sounds and melodies of the music created.

 Visual: Use the eyes to see the instrument, track movement and follow instructions.

 Olfactory: Recognise and become familiar with the smell. Adults may also want to use calming scents, e.g. lavender, to create an ambient setting.

 Gustatory: The taste and sensations in the mouth, particularly when the lips touch and blow brass and wind instruments.

 Interoception: Feel and connect to the internal sensations and vibrations from within the body whilst the music is being created.

 Vestibular: Balance and move the body to play instruments appropriately.

 Proprioceptive: Become aware of how the body is positioned whilst playing the instrument. Help children maintain a comfortable posture.

Therapeutic Games

At the heart of music therapy is the rapport and bond of trust between the music therapist and child, which is developed over time during the session. Alongside professional music therapy, musical interaction games can be used by parents, teachers and other therapists to help children with special needs.

♪♪ Instrumental Conductor

The Instrumental Conductor game is a simple 'call-and-response' type of activity to improve social skills. The conductor (another child or an adult) vocalises or shows visuals to the children to indicate when it's their turn to play their instrument. After a child has played for a short while, the conductor indicates when to stop. For added fun, and depending on the children's level of understanding, exaggerated gestures or additional visuals from the conductor can indicate how to play the instrument: e.g. loud, quietly, fast, slow.

♪♪ Act that Tune

You will need...

- Signs or visuals to show actions

- Pre-recorded sounds (e.g. piano, ocean, birds, lullabies, flutes)

- Musical instruments for live music

- Audio device

This is an attention, listening and cooperation game. A musical story or song is shared with the children – you can ask children to choose a musical story/song they like. Be mindful of the song's desired effect, e.g. use calm music if you would like the children to relax or a more upbeat song to make them more alert. Play the song once or twice with no expectation and allow the children to explore the rhythm and pace.

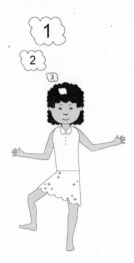

When the children are settled, inform them that the music will play again. This time, whenever the children hear a particular sound or verbal phrase or see a visual cue (depending on the adult's instruction), they create a specific response. Examples of the children's responses could include playing a musical instrument, moving and doing actions with their body, making facial expressions, or singing along to accompany the music. Playing musical movement games like Mirror Your Partner's Actions and Here We Go Round the Mulberry Bush are known to improve 'brain-body neural connections in children which will support their self-regulation development' (Williams, 2014).

In some cases, it may be more appropriate to simply read a short story and ask children to respond whilst listening to the narrative by following visual cues to create sounds or play instruments.

♪♪ Art Expression

You will need...

- Art materials (e.g. paint, pens, clay)
- Paper

- Pre-recorded sounds (e.g. piano, ocean, birds, lullabies, flutes)

- Musical instruments for live music

- Audio device

Listening to music can trigger emotions and memories. These internal sensations may bring children to a state of calm and sense of fulfilment, but, in some cases, music may trigger the memory of unpleasant past experiences. However, once an emotion has been tapped into and recognised, it can be an incredibly healing process towards letting go. Art Expression helps children feel into their emotions whilst expressing creativity.

In preparation, choose live and pre-recorded music from a variety of genres and moods and gather art materials (e.g. glow paint, pens, crayons, clay) and paper. Inform children that when they hear the music they are free to draw, express and create shapes, lines or objects to show how the music makes them feel.

If appropriate, ask the children to choose the music before-hand – discuss their choices and creative efforts before and after the session to reflect on and help process any feelings that may come up. If a child requires hand-over-hand adult support with their fine motor skills, try to ensure the emotive and creative expressions represent the child's feelings.

♫♪ Hot Potato Band

You will need...

- Signs or visuals to show instructions

- Musical instruments (e.g. shaker, bells, rattle anything appropriate)

- Pre-recorded sounds

- Audio device

Musical hot potato is a circle time activity for a small group of children. The game helps develop auditory processing, cognition and social communication skills.

1. Give a shaker, musical rattle, bells or another passable instrument to a child sat within the group circle.

2. Play upbeat or lively music whilst the first child shakes the shaker quickly for 5 seconds, then passes the instrument on to the next child to shake for 5 seconds, who then passes it on around the group.

3. Use visual, verbal or physical support when passing the instrument around the circle, depending on the children's level of understanding.

4. Once everyone has played and passed the instrument around the circle, the game restarts.

5. Continue to play the music and hand the instrument to the first child to shake then pass on. This time round, the music will stop different intervals.

6. When the music stops, the child holding the instrument choose a visual or another instrument from a soft feely bag or similar. The bag usually contains visuals of instructions for children to clap their hands, march on the spot, sing along or tap their feet. Adapt as necessary for your group.

7. Once the child performs the activity, he or she moves to an area just outside the circle (with a supporting adult) to start a 'band'.

8. Restart the music so the rest of the group continue passing the instrument around the circle and child in the 'band' plays along to the music doing the physical actions shown on their visual.

9. Every time the music stops, whoever has the shaker chooses a visual from the feely bag, and moves to join the band. Eventually, the whole group is in the band.

10. The music tends to be upbeat to keep a swift pace,
    however, if the group's pace needs to be slower to calm
    the children, use alternative music that suits the group.

Music offers immense potential to empower and help all children
to breathe, ignite the senses and simply relax. See Animal
Breathing (page 48) and Sound (page 69) for further musical
and sound activities.

Next Steps

The self-regulation activities contained within this chapter can be
adapted to children's cognitive ability, emotional state and therapeutic
needs. Adults may find that children experience the calming benefits
with self-regulation activities on one day and then unexpectedly
find it difficult to settle and self-regulate on other occasions. The
following chapter explores what to do when things do not go to plan
and children require additional support to get started.

Part III

Relax

S — **Stop** what you are doing, gently drop your shoulders and allow yourself to be present in this moment.

T — **Take** some deep breaths as you close your eyes. Focus on your breathing (Chapter 3) and how this gradually helps you feel calm.

A — **And...** Pause for a few moments to observe your thoughts and feelings as you begin to feel more at peace.

R — **Relax**, let go and allow any thoughts and feelings to pass through your mind and body. Take time to gradually gain a more calming state of flow (Chapter 4).

Chapter 5

Positive Strategies

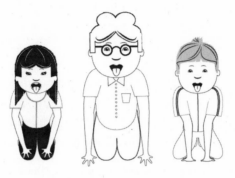

To help children with special needs understand the art of relaxation and the concept of mindfulness, adults need to understand that everything they say and do in front of children is being observed. In many cases, the behaviour of the adults in children's lives gradually forms children's subconscious mind and shapes their beliefs, thoughts and behaviours as they grow into adolescence and adulthood. Therefore, throwaway comments and actions – both good and bad – are being seen and heard by children who often look up to the adults in their lives as role models. Ultimately, adults have a big impact on kids, particularly those with special needs, so when adults are mindful of their behaviour and choice of words, it provides a platform to inspire the special little ones in their life to do the same.

Creating a Safe Space for Relaxation

To help develop a mindful sense of flow and learn to relax, children with special needs need a safe space to feel comfortable in, with the least amount of distractions, as these may trigger overstimulation and anxiety. The key things to consider when finding a suitable space are listed below.

- **Inclusive**: ensure environments are welcoming and respectful, provide inclusive and accessible facilities, are secure, provide a safety net, offer suitable aids appropriate for children's physical, sensory and social needs and create a sense of belonging.

- **Practical**: where possible, provide clearly labelled areas for children to rest, relax and/or have fun in. Examples include chill-out rooms, quiet meditation space, sensory rooms, play areas and private therapy space with calm lighting and sufficient room to move around. Set up practical routines and create visuals and structured boundaries within each environment to help children become familiar with the surroundings, feel safe, develop confidence and navigate their way around with increased independence.

- **Comfort**: comfortable and supportive space and seating is an important aspect to help children feel relaxed. Most notably, lightweight bean bags and therapy exercise balls have been recognised as alternative seating, resulting in children having an increased ability to unwind and concentrate for longer periods of time.

- **Sensory awareness**: become aware of the children's sensory experiences and specific needs to help calm or stimulate children within ambient and/or practical environments and create any adaptations to accommodate them. Work with a therapy team if necessary, because this may involve tailored sensory integration, reduced sensory stimulus, the use of sensory lighting, white wall projectors and appropriate furniture.

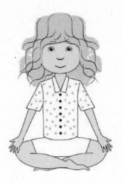

Positive Strategies in Action

As with any activity with children, despite our best efforts, things may not always go to plan. Children with special needs require a high degree of empathy, calm and patience, particularly non-verbal children who are unable to express themselves.

It's important to remember that no child is the same, so consider the diagnoses of the special yogis in your life and feel free to experiment with what works and then adapt any of the activities with appropriate consideration. As you give any instructions, ensure your words, gestures or visual pictorial cues provide simple, calming, step-by-step and clear communication in accordance with the children's understanding and developmental abilities. Remember, for children with special needs, in some cases using the least amount of verbal language is essential because overwhelming amounts of chatter and/or loud tones do not help them feel at ease. Comments like 'First we will sit down, then you can choose a fun breathing activity' provide a simple and direct linguistic approach that can be supported with visual pictorial symbols.

Teaching children how to consciously breathe and use the other self-regulation tools in this book may take time, particularly if they are extremely anxious, accustomed to experiencing meltdowns or feel overwhelmed about a particular situation. Patience, empathy and flexibility are key aspects of working with children with special needs, so give it time and explore using some of the following positive strategies to help children relax.

You will need...

- Visual timetable

- Emotion cards and other emotion visuals (e.g. traffic light think fan)

- Emotions journal

- Calming strategy book or tool box

- Positive behavioural reward system

- Lightweight bean bags and therapy exercise balls

- Sensory integration tools

- Appropriate furniture and chill out space

- Consistent communication between children and all adults

- Make **eye contact** when talking to children, even if they struggle to give direct eye contact themselves. Ensure you have the children's attention by addressing them with their name and/or a gentle touch on the shoulder before talking. When trusted adults attentively look into children's eyes it's likely to make them feel safe and connected and develop feelings of self-worth.

- Establish **consistent routines** with **visual guides** to reassure the children and **set boundaries** and **clear expectations on behaviour**. Be honest, calm and open with the children and, at an appropriate time, **use simple language** to talk through any situations or events when expectations have not been met.

- Break things down by using a **visual timetable** of First, Next, Then/Last to talk the children through the 'baby steps' of each mindfulness activity and show that the expectations are simply to help children feel better about themselves.

- **Scaffold** any of the self-regulation activities you use from this book. First show the children how to practise the mindfulness activity, then ask them to join in and **offer lots of praise** and, lastly, encourage the children to **use the tools independently**.

- Be mindful that in many cases the children may not understand the consequences of their actions or indeed why they behaved in a particular way, so remember to be **fair-minded** and **show empathy**. If appropriate, carefully describe the **Flipping Your Lid** Hand Model on page 143 to help the children understand the reason for their behaviour and adapt your explanation with visuals or simplified language according to the children's understanding.

- **Give the children a choice** of one activity between two or three breathing exercises (use visuals if needed). Alternatively, have children help you create an **emotions journal, calming strategy book** or **strategy tool box** containing visuals, fidget toys to hold or other items that can help them feel calm.

- Connect to the **children's interests** and use role play/guided imagery to **spark their imagination**. Improvise, use visuals if needed and tap into the children's interests. For instance, if a child likes cars, show visuals of cars and replace the sound during the Fish Breath exercise on page 51 to using the 'Vroom Vroom Vroom' sound of a car.

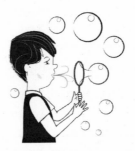

- Allow children '**thinking time**' to process what is being asked of them and don't rush things! Remember, it's perfectly fine for children to step away to a quiet space for a few moments or to go for a walk and then try again with the mindfulness activity.

- Continually **reassure children that everything is okay**, especially for little yogis with perfectionist tendencies. It's alright to make mistakes and feel overwhelmed, angry, frustrated and so forth, as long as they are safe and their actions are not harming others. Remind children that mindfully breathing will help them move through the emotions they are experiencing.

- **Motivate** children to become mindful yogis by giving them lots of praise throughout activities and a choice of rewards to choose between upon completion. Older children may enjoy the responsibility of teaching or **mentoring** their peers or younger children on how to use self-regulation tools.

- Taking a **sensory break** and participating in **physical exercise** like yoga, jumping on a trampoline or crawling along the floor pretending to be an animal can offer children a healthy distraction, lift the tension/emotion out of the body and dispel busy thoughts from the mind. Dr Daniel Siegel and Dr Tina Payne Bryson describe '**Move It Or Lose It**' as a healthy way for the brain to receive calming messages from a physically active body, to return to a state of brain/body integration (Payne Bryson and Siegel, 2015: 52). 'Move It or Lose It' encourages children to physically move their bodies to help improve their mindset. Examples include star jumps, Wall Push Ups (page 93) and Log Rolls (page 89). This form of intervention can be used as a distraction to engage the body and mind towards a more centred and grounded being.

- **Empower children to journal** how they are feeling before and after a situation by drawing a picture, writing about what's troubling them, choosing simple visuals (smiley face/sad face) or talking to a trusted person. Sharing their feelings either verbally or pictorially helps release any angst from within. See the emotions journal in Sections 6 and 7 of Part V: Resources to help children recognise, accept and learn about their emotional state.

- **Develop rapport with children** to **see things from their perspective** and maintain a **supportive connection**. Over time, this can build healthy adult–child relationships and foster children's trust. With good rapport, children become more receptive when adults **show them how to make positive and safe choices,** particularly when feeling overwhelmed.

- Many children with special needs are easily discouraged so continually **celebrate** and **recognise their efforts** to use self-regulation tools. Highlight their strengths and encourage them to appreciate how far they have come to become mindful little yogis.

Flipping Your Lid

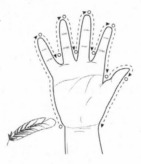

Children's mindfulness practitioners often use Dr Daniel Siegel and Dr Tina Payne Bryson's 'Flipping Your Lid' Hand Model to explain the inner workings of the brain and to encourage children to use self-regulation to help them relax. The Hand Model is a great way to show kids where thoughts, behaviours and emotions come from and how to keep themselves from flipping their lid. Using the hand to demonstrate the brain's actions helps children visualise, label and understand what's going on inside of them. It also encourages children to use self-regulation to change their state and gradually relax.

1. Spread the fingers of one hand out into a star shape.

2. Point to the wrist to explain this represents the spine.

3. Direct children to the palm of the hand, and say the spinal cord comes up into the skull, which first holds the brain stem and limbic area ('downstairs brain').

4. Gently place the thumb on the palm of the hand.

5. The thumb and palm represent the 'downstairs' brain – the area of big emotions, instincts, arousal and the 'alarm centre'.

6. Cover the thumb with the fingers to form a fist shape.

7. The fingers covering the thumb are the 'upstairs' brain – the area of rational thinking, reasoning and perceptions of the outside world.

8. The fist represents the whole brain.

9. Lift the fingers from the thumb and explain that when we get really upset or feel like we've lost control, we 'flip our lid!' because the upstairs, rational, thinking part of the brain is no longer connected to the downstairs, emotional, 'alarm centre' of the brain. If this happens to any of us, we may act out and say or do things we later regret.

10. Lower the fingers to cover the thumb again. Explain that when there is an 'invisible staircase' connecting and regulating the 'upstairs' and 'downstairs' parts of the brain, we still may experience unpleasant feelings and situations, but instead of 'flipping our lid' we can use logical thinking to make the informed choice of practising mindfulness. Using mindful self-regulation activities, e.g. deep breathing, listening to music, etc., tells the brain to help us behave in a much calmer and healthier way.

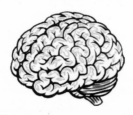

Adapt the instructions above with **simplified language and/or visual symbols** to teach the Hand Model to any children who are cognitively able to understand this information. To simplify this further for low-ability children, an alternative approach would be to **open and close the hands** with less verbal explanation. Open and shake out the hands and fingers to represent overstimulated or heightened emotions and then close both hands into fists to represent calm emotions and a balanced mind-set.

Whenever children feel stressed or overwhelmed, remind them to look down at their hands, close their fingers over the thumb and answer the question: 'What do you think the "upstairs" part of your brain wants to tell the "downstairs" part of your brain to help you feel calm?' By responding to this question and progressing through some of the mindful self-regulation tools from Chapter 3 onwards, children can learn how to self-regulate by rationally containing their emotions and feeling more grounded. For more information on the inner workings of the upstairs and downstairs brain, refer to page 102.

Due to the differing needs and emotions that arise in children on any given day, instilling mindfulness tools and positive strategies can take time. Remember to be flexible, creative, calm and, most importantly, patient. Teaching children how to relax and self-regulate by connecting to the breath and developing a sense of flow is a gradual process. However, with consistent practice, setting clear boundaries and developing routines can make all the difference.

Part IV

Final Reflections

S **Stop** what you are doing, gently drop your shoulders and allow yourself to be present in this moment.

T **Take** some deep breaths as you close your eyes. Focus on your breathing (Chapter 3) and how this gradually helps you feel calm.

A **And...** Pause for a few moments to observe your thoughts and feelings as you begin to feel more at peace.

R **Relax**, let go and allow any thoughts and feelings to pass through your mind and body. Take time to gradually gain a more calming state of flow (Chapter 4).

Conclusion

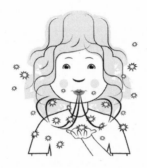

Mindful Little Yogis is a book derived from research-based theories, pedagogy and ancient spiritual philosophies. Carefully written to inspire children from all walks of life and with all abilities, especially those with special needs, to practice mindfulness, this book can be used in a variety of educational, therapeutic and casual settings. With the continued practice of the self-regulation tools contained within *Mindful Little Yogis*, belief systems can be transformed, creating mindful behaviours with children's lives reshaped towards becoming empowered individuals armed with a bank of calming strategies to get through each day.

Chapter 1 explored the world of special education needs (SEN), the modern-day classroom and how mindfulness and yoga philosophies help children process life's ups and downs. This chapter also highlighted four main areas of the *Special Educational Needs and Disability Code of Practice: 0 to 25 Years* (Department for Education, 2015) in England – namely cognition and learning; social, emotional and mental health; communication and interaction; and sensory and/or physical needs – as the key aspects that children with special needs require support with, providing informed guidance for the content of this book. Chapter 2 showed us the S.T.A.R. model, a simple step-by-step approach for kids and adults to use as a guide as they progress through the activities in this book. By repeatedly learning and practising self-regulation strategies with the S.T.A.R. model, children develop new behavioural habits due to the creation of neuropathways in the brain to reinforce the use of mindful calming strategies, particularly during times of heightened emotions. Chapters 3 and 4 reminded us that everything starts with the breath and provided an extensive range of practical self-regulation strategies, including animal breathing, chanting, keeping an emotions journal and practising sensory yoga. Chapter 5 detailed positive strategies to help children relax and feel empowered when applying the self-regulation tools in this book, particularly as introducing new activities to children with special needs can take time and requires a high degree of patience, flexibility and empathy. And lastly, the following section contains supporting resources for readers to use alongside the main content of this book.

To reemphasise a point mentioned in Chapter 2, the content of *Mindful Little Yogis* is adaptable. Depending on your circumstances and the children, things will undoubtedly change, so whilst using the S.T.A.R. model to incorporate mindfulness, it's perfectly acceptable to adjust and accommodate activities for the special little children in your life where necessary. However, it's also important to have fun, so enjoy the process!

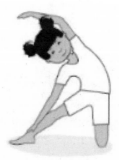

Whilst reflecting on the use of *Mindful Little Yogis*, readers are encouraged to think about their own experience of participating in the activities within this book. Self-reflection and mindfulness go hand in hand. Granted, mindfulness is about connecting to the present moment, paying attention without judgement and living in the here and now, whereas self-reflection involves looking back at previous events to help individuals question themselves in a positive way, bringing a renewed perspective into the present moment. Self-reflection enables us to review and celebrate the things that went well, recognise the things that didn't go so well, explore opportunities to improve and move forward with a renewed perspective.

You are now invited to reflect upon the impact this book has had on you and the little yogis in your life. To self-reflect consider:

- the self-regulation activities that the children particularly enjoyed

- your lightbulb moments and the activities you enjoyed the most

- any challenges experienced and how you overcame them

- the sorts of things you had to change or simplify to make things more accessible

- the types of places the exercises worked well in and the places to avoid in future

- the times of day the children were more receptive to using the tools

- any feelings that came up for you whilst helping the children, compared with how you feel now

- how these mindfulness activities have helped you and the children you work or live with

- whether, after regular practice and modelling mindfulness, you have begun to see a difference in your child's behaviour and emotional state.

Mindfully explore your reflections and connect to how this makes you feel and the difference you have made to the children you support. Share your reflections and exchange ideas with other similar parents, therapists or educators. By doing this, you may just inspire yourself and others to make a difference to the lives of even more children. Information sharing creates a network of potentially supportive like-minded adults that help expand ideas to encourage more children and adults to practice mindfulness.

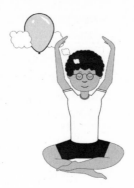

Mindful Little Yogis is exactly what you make it. The content can be viewed as a handy 'go-to' text to dip into every day as part of a routine for fun and inspiring self-regulation tools to help the special kids in your life or as a practical reference tool to use whenever the children you live or work with are finding it difficult to cope with life's ups and down. The choice is yours. Either way, every child is different, and each activity will need to be mindfully approached with empathy to ensure the children feel completely supported and are able to gain access to self-regulation tools in accordance with their needs.

Showing children how to calm down and use self-regulation tools doesn't have to be perfect – just getting started and focusing on the breath is key! Whilst using this book, adults may become more conscious of their own breathing and other self-regulation activities. This in turn gradually develops a mindful outlook on renewed ways to creatively empower children to become the best version of themselves, resulting in positive, long-term changes to enhance the mental and emotional well-being of children.

The most meaningful element for children to see and experience in their young lives is when the adults they trust and look up to consistently use mindfulness to deal with life's daily ups and downs. This is particularly true for children who are prone to meltdowns, anxiety, overwhelm and confusion. When adults promote mindful-ness by being present in each moment, consciously breathing and showing kindness to themselves and others, they develop a sense of compassion, empathy and gratitude. To this end, when children observe adults' mindful actions, words and behaviours and the impact this has on their lives, it encourages them to eventually seek and learn healthier ways to relax, self-regulate, develop a more grounded approach towards life and be less disheartened when things don't go to plan. This can take time, as every day may come with a new challenge. Buddha once said, 'It is during our darkest moments that we must focus to see the light.' In essence, this book aims to equip you with the tools to shine your inner light and ignite the light of the special little yogis in your life. **Namaste** ♥

Part V

Resources

Developmental Skills Glossary

Auditory discrimination: Auditory discrimination is a child's ability to differentiate between sounds by identifying which words/sounds are similar and distinguishing the difference between words/sounds.

Body awareness: Body awareness is the sense a child has over their own body. With body awareness a child is able to understand the different parts of his or her body, where their body parts are located, how they feel and what their body parts can do.

Cognitive learning or cognitive development: Cognitive ability is a child's ability to learn and process information. Cognitive learning/development is developed through the thought processes of problem-solving, remembering details, recalling information on and making informed decisions.

Crossing the body's midline: Imagine an invisible line centred vertically down the middle of the body. Crossing the midline is a child's ability to use their arms and/or legs to reach across to the other side of their body. An example would be the right elbow touching the left knee or placing the left hand on the right ear.

Fine motor: Fine motor is the child's ability to use the small muscles in the hands, fingers, and tongue. Fine motor skills are used during drawing, eating, cutting with scissors and tying shoe laces.

Gross motor: Gross motor is a child's ability to use large muscles in the body. Gross motor examples include sitting, crawling and running.

Hand–eye coordination: Hand–eye coordination is achieved when a child uses their vision to move and coordinate their hands with a degree of control. Examples include catching a ball, handwriting or picking up an object with the hands.

Oral motor: Oral motor is a child's ability to use the lips, cheeks, tongue and jaw to perform any activity involving oral skills, particularly when eating, talking and breathing through the mouth.

Organisation skills: Organisation is a child's ability to prepare themselves for a task by understanding what is involved, gathering any materials required and then following instructions or using their previous experience to complete the task.

Phonological awareness: Phonological awareness is a child's ability to focus on, discriminate and use specific sounds (phonemes) to create spoken words.

Planning and sequencing: Planning and sequencing is a child's ability to follow the sequences of a task to achieve a defined outcome. This can be anything from brushing the teeth to putting clothes on.

Visual perception: Visual perception is a child's ability to use the brain to make sense of what the eyes can see.

Visual tracking: Visual tracking is a child's ability to use the eyes to focus on a moving object within their immediate vision. This is the eyes' ability to fluidly move up and down, from left to right or in circular motions to keep track of an object.

Self-care: Self-care is a child's ability to develop skills to look after themselves. Examples include washing the face, eating and putting shoes on.

Stimulate the senses: To stimulate a child's senses is to awaken and arouse one or more of the eight senses. The sensory systems are gustatory (taste), tactile (touch), olfactory (smell), visual (sight), auditory (sound), vestibular (movement and balance), proprioceptive (body awareness) and interoceptive (internal bodily sensations).

Bubble (Circle) Reading

Read the bubbles like a story!

Every time you see a big bubble, take a deep breath in and slow breath out.

Every time you see a little bubble, take a small breath in and quick breath out.

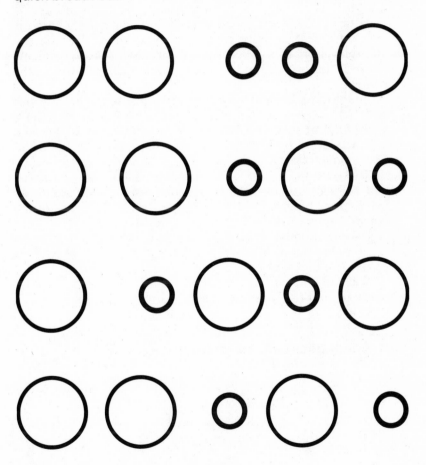

Have fun and colour each bubble in!

My name is: _____

SECTION 3

Guided Imagery Scripts

Part 1: Starfish Guided Imagery

The children should sit or lie down with their backs straight and arms gently resting on the body.

Read this script slowly and calmly:

> Close your eyes. Take a slow, deep breath in through the nose. Breathe out slowly through the mouth. Feel the muscles in your body. Continue to breathe in and out deeply through your nose. Notice the breath taking you deeper and deeper into relaxation. Every muscle in your body is feeling calm and relaxed. This is your time to feel at peace. Continue to breathe deeply.
>
> Imagine you are a starfish floating in the ocean and this feels so good. Move your legs and arms gently just like a peaceful starfish. Deeply breathe in as you take your arms and legs apart and breathe out to bring them back to the body. Feel yourself floating.
>
> The ocean is a calming shade of blue. As you go deeper and deeper, you see different colours, hear sounds, see other fish happily floating and can smell the clear freshness of the ocean. Feel the light energy enter your body.
>
> Deeply breathe in as you take your arms and legs apart and breathe out to bring them back to the body. Feel yourself continuing to float.
>
> You can return to the ocean whenever you want to. Now be ready to continue your day feeling happy and at ease.
>
> Open your eyes when you are ready. Well done!

Part 2: Sun Bliss Guided Imagery

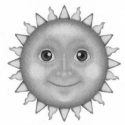

The children should sit or lie down with their backs straight and arms gently resting on the body.

Read this script slowly and calmly:

Close your eyes. Take a slow, deep breath in through the nose. Breathe out slowly through the mouth. Feel the muscles in your body. Continue to breathe in and out deeply through your nose. Notice the breath taking you deeper and deeper into relaxation. Every muscle in your body is feeling calm and relaxed. This is your time to feel at peace. Continue to breathe deeply.

Imagine you are walking in a park and see a small pond surrounded by trees. There are swans floating peacefully across the water. You head towards the pond and can see your face reflected back in the water. Breathe in as you smile at your reflection. Breathe out as you continue to smile.

The sky is blue and the sun is shining. This fills you with calm and peaceful energy. Breathe in the calming, peaceful energy from the blue sky, and breathe out any cloudy feelings. Continue to breathe in and breathe out deeply.

The sun is warming up the water, swans, trees, grass and everything in the park. Your body is feeling warm and there's a lovely gentle breeze. As you breathe in you smile again and as you deeply breathe out you continue to feel blissful.

Imagine the sun's gentle warmth entering and spreading through your entire body. The sun's warm energy flows from your face to your neck, then to your chest, down into the belly and into your entire back. Continue to breathe and absorb this cleansing energy from your shoulders down the arms to your fingertips. Imagine that warm feeling now spreading into your hips and down to both legs and, lastly, from the feet towards your toes.

The sunlight rays have created such a warm, peaceful and calming feeling in your whole body. Keep breathing. You can return to this park whenever you want to. Now be ready to continue your day feeling calm and blissful.

Open your eyes when you are ready. Well done!

Grounding with Progressive Relaxation

The children should lie down or sit in a comfortable position with their backs straight. If they are seated, ensure both feet are placed flat on the ground.

Read this script slowly and calmly:

Take in some deep breaths. Slowly inhale and exhale. You begin to feel your body relax from the top of your head to the tips of your toes. Continue to feel the breath coming to your nose as your belly moves up and down at the same time as your breath.

Notice how your breath feels. Notice how your body feels. We are now going to focus on parts of your body.

Start with your feet. Breathe in as you curl in your toes and squeeze the muscles in your feet. Breathe out to release the muscles.

Now gently sway both legs. As you breathe in squeeze the muscles in your left leg, then breathe out to release the muscles. Relax. As you breathe in squeeze the muscles in your right leg, then breathe out to release the muscles. Imagine your legs are now strings of spaghetti – all floppy and relaxed. Bring the energy back into your legs by continuing to breathe naturally.

Now wriggle your fingers. As you breathe in make a fist and squeeze your left hand. Breathe out to open your left hand. As you breathe in make a fist and squeeze your right hand. Breathe out to open your right hand. Imagine you have just squeezed all the juice out of an orange with your hands and now relax. Continue to breathe deeply.

Now gently move your arms. As you breathe in squeeze the left arm and lift the left shoulder. Breathe out to release all the muscles in this arm and shoulder. Relax. Breathe in to squeeze the right arm and lift the right shoulder. Breathe out to release the muscles in this arm. Relax. Breathe in and gently raise both hands and arms above the head. Image a fluffy cloud peacefully floating above you. Breathe in and breathe out. Breathe in. Breathe out as you release the arms back down to the sides of the body feeling light and at ease. Feeling so relaxed. Notice how you feel.

Now focus on the belly moving up and down with your breathing. Breathe in to squeeze and gently push the belly out, then breathe out to let the muscles release. Breathe in to gently push the belly out, then breathe out to let the muscles release. Imagine this is a balloon letting out all the air.

Now notice your face and how this feels. Relax. Breathe in to scrunch up your nose, cheeks, lips, mouth, forehead and eyes as much as you can. Breathe out to let go.

Your whole body is now relaxed and peaceful. Notice how this feels to let go. Continue to breathe deeply. This is your time to relax for a few moments.

Now, in your own time, slowly open your eyes feeling so calm and relaxed. Well done!

Yoga Story Script

To prepare children for this story, initially read the script two or three times out loud from the left side of the table without the physical yoga actions. Then read the story again and incorporate the yoga poses and actions. Be mindful not to read the actions part (right side of table) of the story to the children – this is only for adult reference.

Yoga Story: Josie the Star ॐ

Yoga Story Script (verbally communicated by the adult to children)	Yoga poses and movements alongside the story (children respond by mirroring the adult's physical actions and sounds)
Josie loves to relax.	Sit in cross legged pose (Sukhasana). Breathe in and out deeply (Pranayama).
To help her feel calm, she likes to chant: 'Peace begins with me. Peace begins with me. Peace begins with me.'	Chant along to 'Peace begins with me.'
Josie looks through her yoga goggles.	Place the finger and thumb of each hand to touch each other (Gyana Mudra). Look through the space in between the finger and thumb (yoga goggles) with the eyes. Turn the head and upper body left, right, up and down with the body still seated.
She can see a big, tall mountain with a shiny, big star at the top of the mountain.	Slowly stand up and move the body into mountain pose (Tadasana).
Josie decides to climb up the mountain to find the star.	Gently walk on the spot or up and down the yoga mat.
On her way up the mountain, Josie hears a bumble bee buzzing with a humming sound. She greets the bee by humming back to it.	Take a deep breath, exhale by humming through the nose and place the index fingers over the ear lobes (Bhramari Pranayama). Repeat three times.

The bee smiles at Josie and flies away.	Look up, smile and wave.
Josie carries on walking but can now hear a dog barking.	Move into downward dog pose (Adho Mukha Svānāsana) and breathe deeply. If appropriate, make the sound of a barking dog.
Josie realises the dog is chasing a cat. Oh dear!	Move into cat pose (Marjaryasana). Make the sound of a cat meowing.
The cat doesn't look happy. He looks sad and quite scared of the dog.	Return to cross legged pose (Sukhasana). Make a sad face for five seconds and then a scared face for five seconds.
Josie wants to help the cat so she looks through her yoga goggles.	Place the finger and thumb of each hand to touch each other (Gyana Mudra). Look through the space in between the finger and thumb (yoga goggles) with the eyes. Turn the head and upper body left, right, up and down with the body still seated.
Josie can see a big, tall tree near the top of the mountain.	Slowly stand up and move into tree pose (Vrksasana). Make sure this posture is done on both sides. Return to mountain pose (Tadasana).
Josie bends down to pick up the cat and then quietly hides the poor thing behind the tree. She waves goodbye to the cat who is now smiling.	Gently move into standing forward bend (Uttanasana). Return to mountain pose (Tadasana), look down and wave.
Josie looks up and is so happy because she is now at the top of the mountain. She can see, feel, hear and touch the big, bright, sparkly star!	Position the body into a five-pointed star (Utthita Tadasana).
She decides to celebrate and show gratitude for reaching the top of the mountain.	Do five star jumps and make a cheer sound at the end.

Josie reminds herself that she is a very brave and kind girl, who will always allow her special, star-like qualities to shine from within.	Hug and squeeze your own shoulders and upper arms for a few moments. If it's appropriate, the children can also hug the adult and/or their peers.
Now it's time to have a peaceful rest and settle down with a relaxed body and calm mind.	Slowly and gently lay down on the back with the arms beside the body and a straight back (Savasana). Breathe deeply.

Calming Strategy Visual

Things that help me feel calm...

Rectangle: Draw or stick in a picture of yourself.

Circles: Draw the things that help you feel calm.

This is ME:

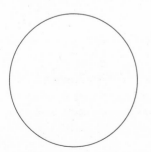

My name is: _____

SECTION 7

Faces of Emotion

Draw these faces.

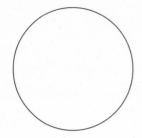

I feel sad

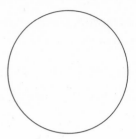

I feel happy

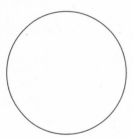

I feel scared

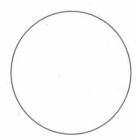

I feel excited

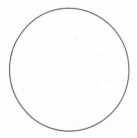

I feel angry

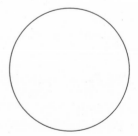

I feel sleepy

My name is: _____

References

Baptiste, B. (2016) *Perfectly Imperfect: The Art and Soul of Yoga Practice*. Carlsbad, CA: Hay House.

Baron-Cohen, S., Gomez, G., Krauss, G. and LeGoff, D. (2014) *Lego®-Based Therapy*. London: Jessica Kingsley Publishers.

Cicchetti, D., Ganiban, J. and Barnett, D. (1991) 'Contributions from the Study of High-Risk Populations to Understanding the Development of Emotion Regulation.' In J. Garber and K. A. Dodge (eds) *Cambridge Studies in Social and Emotional Development. The Development of Emotion Regulation and Dysregulation* (pp.15–48). Cambridge: Cambridge University Press.

Collins, B. (2015) *Sensory Yoga for Kids: Therapeutic Movement for Children of All Abilities*. Arlington, TX: Sensory World.

Department for Education (2015) *Special Educational Needs and Disability Code of Practice: 0 to 25 years*. London: Department for Education.

Drinkwater-Burke, B. (2016) *LEGO® Therapy*. CD-ROM.

Harvard Medical School (2018) *How Music Can Help You Heal*. Accessed on 12/03/2018 at: www.health.harvard.edu/mind-and-mood/how-music-can-help-you-heal.

Hughes, E. (2017) *The Go Yogi! Card Set*. London: Singing Dragon.

Kabat-Zinn, J. (2004) *Wherever You Go, There You Are*. London: Piatkus Books Ltd.

Ofsted (2010) *The Special Educational Needs and Disability Review*. Manchester: Ofsted.

Oxford University Press (2015) *English Oxford Living Dictionaries*. Accessed on 20/02/2018 at: https://en.oxforddictionaries.com/definition/mindfulness.

Payne Bryson, T. and Siegel, D. (2012) *The Whole Brain Child*. London: Robinson.

Payne Bryson, T. and Siegel, D. (2015) *The Whole Brain Child Workbook*. Eau Claire, WI: PESI Publishing and Media.

Sanger, K. L. and Dorjee, D. (2015) 'Mindfulness training for adolescents: A neuro-developmental perspective on investigating modifications in attention and emotion regulation using event-related brain potentials.' *Cognitive, Affective and Behavioral Neuroscience 15*, 3, 696–711.

Williams, K. (2014) *Early Childhood Self-Regulation Through Music*. The Early Childhood Researcher. Accessed on 21/02/2018 at: www.theearlychildhoodresearcher.wordpress.com/2014/12/10/early-childhood-self-regulation-through-music.

Further Reading

Amor, J. (2013) *Five Fun Breathing Exercises for Kids.* Accessed on 20/02/2018 at www.cosmickids.com/read/five-fun-breathing-practices-for-kids.

Bates, W. (1920) *The Cure of Imperfect Sight Without Glasses.* New York: Central Fixation Publishing Co.

Brown, R. and Gerbarg, P. (2009) *Yoga Breathing, Meditation, and Longevity.* New York: Columbia University College of Physicians and Surgeons.

British Association of Music Therapy *What is Music Therapy?* Accessed on 21/02/2018 at: www.bamt.org/music-therapy/what-is-music-therapy.html.

Chaplin, B. and Penner, M. (2012) *Helping Young People Learn Self-Regulation.* Chapin, SC: Youth Light Inc.

Chevalier, G., Ober, C. and Zucker, M. (2015) *Grounding the Human Body: The Healing Benefits of Earthing.* The Chopra Center. Accessed on 20/02/2018 at: www.chopra.com/articles/grounding-the-human-body-the-healing-benefits-of-earthing#sm.00005ysk wx9gnf0xsim2o3clnxymp.

Copeland, L. (1998) *Hunter and His Amazing Remote Control: A Fun, Hands-On Way to Teach Self-Control to ADD/ADHD Children.* Chapin, SC: Youth Light Inc.

Garrigan, N. (2014) *Rainbow Breathing Exercise and Worksheet.* Accessed on 20/02/2018 at: http://branchhabitat.blogspot.co.uk/2014/03/rainbow-breathing-exercise-and-worksheet.html.

GoNoodle, Get Moving (2016) *Rainbow Breath – Flow Video.* Accessed on 21/02/2018 at: www.youtube.com/watch?v=O29e4rRMrV4.

Harvard University Research (2017) *Executive Function and Self-Regulation.* Cambridge, MA: Center on the Developing Child at Harvard University. Accessed on 20/02/2018 at: https://developingchild.harvard.edu/science/key-concepts/executive-function.

Iyengar, B. K. S. (2002) *Light on the Yoga Sutras of Patanjali.* London: Thorsons Publishing Group.

Laurent, C., Prizant, B., Rubin, E. and Wetherby, A. (2003) 'The SCERTS Model: A transactional, family-centered approach to enhancing communication and socioemotional abilities of children with autism spectrum disorder.' *Infants and Young Children 16,* 4, 296–231.

LeBlanc, M. (2016) *Engaging Breathing Exercises for Children.* Yogi Frogz. Accessed on 20/02/2018 at: www.yogifrogzkids.com/2016/03/10/engaging-breathing-excercises-for-children.

Lender, H. (2013) *Kidding Around Yoga Teacher Training Manual.* Florida: Kidding Around Yoga Publishing.

Mitchell, J. (2017) *Mindfulness: Fad or Business Tool?* Accessed on 20/02/2018 at: www. linkedin.com/pulse/mindfulness-fad-business-tool-joshua-mitchell-mba-ma/?tracki ngId=qww5694oQMmVpYP7TqzUnw%3D%3D.

Moules, J. (2015) *How to Teach Kids 5 Pranayama Breathing Techniques.* YogiApproved.com: Your Life On and Off the Mat. Accessed on 21/02/2018 at: www.yogiapproved.com/ yoga/how-to-teach-kids-5-pranayama-breathing-techniques.

Nhat Hanh, T. (2011) *Planting Seeds: Practicing Mindfulness with Children (Five-Finger Meditation: Mike Bell (pp. 87–88)).* Berkeley, CA: Parallax Press.

Sentis Online Videos (2012) *Neuroplasticity in the Brain.* Accessed on 21/02/2018 at: www. youtube.com/watch?v=ELpfYCZa87g,

Siegel, D. (2012) *Presenting a Hand Model of the Brain Video.* FtMyersFamPsych. Accessed on 21/02/2018 at: www.youtube.com/watch?v=gm9CIJ74Oxw.

Sridhar, V. (2015) *What is Mindfulness?* Ekhart Yoga. Accessed on 21/02/2018 at: www. ekhartyoga.com/articles/what-is-mindfulness.

YoungMinds (2018) *Looking After Yourself: Take Time Out.* Accessed on 21/02/2018 at: www.youngminds.org.uk/find-help/looking-after-yourself/take-time-out.

Index